AF413322

Art of Writing & Publishing in Pharmaceutical Journals

Second Edition

Art of Writing & Publishing in Pharmaceutical Journals
Second Edition

Ajay Semalty

M. Pharm., MBA, Ph. D., PDF (Japan)

Course Coordinator- industrial Pharmacy-I (SWAYAM MOOC)

Assistant Professor,

Department of Pharmaceutical Sciences,

H.N.B. Garhwal University (A Central University)

Srinagar (Garhwal), Uttarakhand

Visiting Scientist

Faculty of Pharmacy, Meijo University Nagoya, Japan

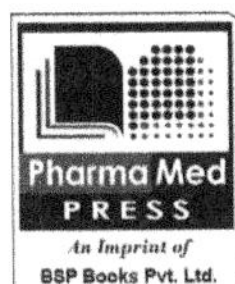

PharmaMed Press

An imprint of BSP Books pvt. Ltd

4-4-309/316, Giriraj Lane,

Sultan Bazar, Hyderabad - 500 095.

Art of Writing & Publishing in Pharmaceutical Journals, *Second edition* *by Ajay Semalty*

© 2022 *by Author*

Published by

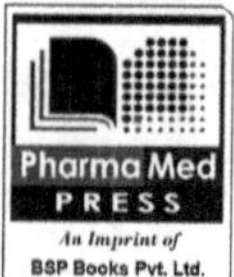

PharmaMed Press

An imprint of BSP Books Pvt. Ltd.
4-4-309/316, Giriraj Lane, Sultan Bazar, Hyderabad - 500 095.
Phone: 040-23445688; Fax: 91+40-23445611
e-mail: info@pharmamedpress.com
www.pharmamedpress.com/pharmamedpress.net

Printed at
Repro India Limited.

Price: Rs. 395.00
ISBN: 978-93-91910-34-1 (Paerback)

Contents

SECTION II
Thesis/ Dissertation Execution & Writing

APPENDIX 1

APPENDIX 2

APPENDIX 3

APPENDIX 4

APPENDIX 5

SECTION I
Paper Writing

CHAPTER 1

Paper Publications in Academic Career

The paper publication is an utmost requirement of an academic and research career. It is the way to communicate your hard work effectively with the global academic and researcher fraternity. An academician or researcher always feels proud of his or her publications and is given due recognition. The publications may of several types.

Types and Traits of academic writing

Paper publication is one of the types of academic writing. In academics, it is a well-established trend and responsibility to share our gathered knowledge via writing an essay, passages, dissertation, thesis, research/ review articles, short notes, books, abstract, digital writing/ OERs etc.

Basic requirements and steps of academic writing

For all types of writing, the basic traits are the same.

- Critical reading: The first and foremost step of the academic writing process is critical reading. In this process, the reader gets engaged with the text deeply and in a complex manner. This engagement promotes readers' critical questioning with the context of the text. It also develops the understanding of judgment about the mechanism of effective communication. In reading, we just absorb the idea or understand it, while in critical reading, we go through analysis, interpretation, and evaluation. Another difference between reading and critical reading is that in reading, our direction of understanding is towards the direction of the text while in critical reading, our direction is just opposite as we try to question every assumption and argument available. After reading, we conclude the text as a summary, but we interpret and describe the text in the case of critical reading.

- Language: Language is the second important part of academic writing. The most exciting fact about language is that your doing with language (output) reflects the language you have absorbed (input). So to write better, you have to read the best. Reading the academic write-ups is the first step in the process of writing. Learning one language is a different thing than getting that language into our awareness. Academic writing requires awareness of the language.

- Good knowledge of grammar, vocabulary, and mechanics is also the central part of academic writing, which clearly demonstrates our ideas in a sophisticated and precise way.

- The clarity: In all forms of writing, you must be very clear in communicating your idea to the reader.

- Completeness: Each communication should be complete in totality. We can not leave it open-ended like in literature.

- Rational & Logic: The rational and logic must be there

- Technicality: Technical terms are always used depending on the field of research.

- Sequencing: The sequence of presenting the information is crucial for a smooth transition from one point to the next point. Connecting ideas and a cohesive writing style is a prime requirement in academic writing.

- Unambiguity: There is no place for ambiguity in AW.

- The reader friendliness is the key point.

In every kind of academic writing, the purpose of writing should be argumentary. The academic credibility of content is very important.

The process of academic writing consists of the following steps. Each step has its significance, and it is necessary to be followed cautiously (Table 1).

Table 1 Flow of action in AW

Step One Generating Ideas		Step Two Generating Outlines	Step Three Writing the First Draft	Step Four Writing Multiple Draft	Step Five Writing Final Draft	Step Six Publishing
Critical Reading	Critical Thinking					
• Analyze • Evaluate	• Interpret • Literature review	• Build framework around the idea • Sequencing of idea and sub-idea	• Flexible ideas • Revising outline • Visual representation • Listing sources	• Revision of write-up • Major changes • Feedback	• Formatting the final write-up • Proofreading	• Follow-up publishers guideline

The importance of AW

If we split the importance concerning importance for stakeholders, the different stakeholders may have different points of importance.

For academicians

If you are a teacher, you might be well aware of the importance of publications. Can you imagine an academician without publications? I think this simple question is itself the answer. Just to list out, for teachers, the publication is

- an effective and well-accepted medium to disseminate the knowledge: Apart from your classroom teaching, if you go for publications, you will reach to more learners and students and will be able to disseminate your knowledge globally. So why be local be global.

- A tool for assessing the eligibility for new academic/ research positions or promotions: All institutions give huge weightage to publications for recruiting and promoting faculty members. For this, you all know that the quality publications published in reputed journals play a vital role. UGC regulation 2018 provides points for publications as Academic Performance Indicator (API).

- A benchmark to assess academic proficiency: Without any access to an academician's CV, the publications are always reliable indicators of their expertise. For example, do you get the reviewer's invitation from reputed journals? If yes, indeed, you might be having a good publication record in that area of research.

- A tool of Intellectual contribution to the knowledge domain: The teacher is ought to give a significant intellectual contribution to the knowledge domain. Even if you are not an active researcher you need to write to contribute in learning process. So, why do you want to limit yourself to your few students? Come up and contribute.

How good you are as a teacher is generally assessed and approved by your publications.

For students:

In this digital era students hardly go for writing lecture notes or some other basic writing. So, when it comes to deliver a piece of AW it becomes a hurricane task for them. Then students start putting the efforts. So, do not just wait for the last moment for delivering. Practice by preparing concise, logical, to the point and quality notes whatever you have been taught in the class. Furthermore, always get it checked or reviewed by your mentor. For students the academic writing is important for getting these vital benefits.

- **Opens up your mind:** When you write your brain works more effectively and new areas of brain start working. Learning to read and write alters brain wiring within months, even for adults

- **Better understanding of the topic for effective communication:** If you know AW you can effectively express or communicate your level of understanding.

- **Triggering the analytical thinking:** AW trigger the analytical thinking. Furthermore, being analytical is important for academic and research. You are required to analytically study two or more related studies for getting the essence out of the work as your future plan of work. You are ought to study and present two or more work analytically rather than doing simple description of previous works.

- **Triggering critical and objective thinking:** Learning is not complete until it is thought critically and objectively. Without critical thinking information can not be framed to build knowledge. (Information□ Knowledge□ Wisdom)

- **Learning Focused and framed writing:** As you have to be more formal and bound to some framework or style in AW. It enables you to deliver the best in the required style/template/framework (as per the requirement of thesis/articles etc).

- **Fulfilling the mandatory requirement:** In the PG dissertations and Ph D thesis, papers are mandatory requirement for submission.

For researchers

If you are a researcher, publication is very vital and indispensable for you. Let see, why it is important.

- **Getting your work evaluated for free:** Can you get your research work evaluated with peers without any cost of time and money? Just write a paper communicate to a good journal. Even if your paper is rejected you will get the vital inputs, comments and suggestions from the experts FOR FREE. Moreover, you will find that many a times even your supervisor can't give these vital suggestions.

- **Fulfilling the mandatory requirement of publications with Ph D thesis:** Almost in all institutions published articles out of the work are to be submitted for getting the permission to submit Ph D thesis.

- **Sharing the research output with national and international researchers:** you publish your work in reputed journals and by this you present your work (in the form of research or review articles etc.) globally.

- **Getting recognition/ international approval for your work:** When you publish a paper, it is evident that it has gone through the rigorous peer-review process from the experts of the field. So it is itself recognition as well as the international approval of your work.

- **Giving weight to your CV and getting weightage in the academic and research jobs:** publications are the heart of a researcher's CV. This gives an immediate impression of your proficiency in research. Author metric like h index, total citations etc gives direct message to the world how effective a researcher you are…. We will discuss these in next week's chapters.

- **Planning future research:** AW lays a foundation for future work. When you plan, design and draft a manuscript at that time only you will find that this this point are to be kept in mind in future while doing the experiments. Alternatively, you will be able to chalk out the next level of work for further stage of your research.

- **Getting project grants:** Only when you have the prior publications on the field of your project proposal you have the chances to get the grants from funding agencies.

For Institutions

- **As Performance indicator of Institutions:** Many well known agencies do the survey and use number of publications and citations to measure performance for their ranking. Times higher education world university ranking (www.thewur.com) ranks global institutions on the basis of several factors including total number of publications by the institutes. In national level, India has a similar ranking of institutions through the National Institutional Ranking Framework (NIRF). (https://www.nirfindia.org/2018/Ranking2018.html). All institutes showcase their total number of publications on their website's homepage to show their excellence in research.

- **For getting the funds from funding agencies:** After patents and technology development, almost all the institutes give prime importance to AW. The one who performs well gets more funds from government agencies or has better chances to get funds.

- Attracting Prospective students, Researchers and foreign collaborations
- Publications of an institute are the marker of its reliability as state of art research institute. This helps to attract prospective students, researchers and foreign collaborators. The collaborations further take the research to the next level and give recognition globally.
- Building goodwill and prestige: Directly or indirectly, it also builds goodwill of the institute in the academic, society and market. This helps in attracting more campus placement of students.

Challenges

We have discussed a lot about the importance and positive side of the publications. Nevertheless, let us have a look on the challenges or other side of the coin. Knowingly or unknowingly, many authors or researchers are indulged in unethical publication practices. Ghostwriting, publishing in substandard journals, contract writing, falsification, fabrication, plagiarism, paid publication etc. are some of the unethical practices which must be avoided to preserve academic integrity. The focus of publications must be on quality and not quantity. In the Indian context, the flood of TDH (Tom Dick and Harry) journals has also affected the credibility of Indian research globally. To get more and more score in Academic performance indicators, many researchers are just publishing for numbers.

Please remember the trend has come that many states of art institutes and Universities just ask for the papers published in SCI-indexed journals. Then all your efforts and money to publish your papers and to have a long list of papers in those TDH journals will go all in vain.

We must not fall in the trap of these TDH journals just to increase the numbers. Publishing in these substandard journals may be disgraceful for authors and their institutes.

Suggested Readings

- https://www.nirfindia.org/2018/Ranking2018.html
- https://www.timeshighereducation.com/
- The best universities in the world 2019, https://www.youtube.com/watch?v=9GNVbF140F8
- The Handbook of Academic Writing: A Fresh Approach By Rowena Murray; Sarah Moore Open University Press, 2006

References

- Faber J, Writing scientific manuscripts: most common mistakes, Dental Press J Orthod. 2017; 22(5): 113–117. doi: 10.1590/2177-6709.22.5.113-117.sar

- Ohwovoriole AE, Writing biomedical manuscripts part I: fundamentals and general rules.West Afr J Med. 2011 May-Jun;30(3):151-7.

- Ohwovoriole AE, West Afr J Med. Writing biomedical manuscripts part II: standard elements and common errors. 2011 Nov-Dec;30(6):389-99.

- https://www.nytimes.com/2014/06/19/science/researching-the-brain-of-writers.html

- Gwendolyn Bounds, How Handwriting Trains the Brain, Oct 5, 2010; https://www.wsj.com/articles/SB10001424052748704631504575531932754922518#articleTabes%3Darticle

- Nature News, Nature, 2018: doi: 10.1038/d41586-018-00927-4

- Nature News, Nature; 2016: doi:10.1038/nature.2016.19198

- Nature News, Nature; 2014: doi:10.1038/nature.2014.14684

- arxiv.org/abs/1707.01162 : Publish Or Impoverish: An investigation of the monetary reward system of science in China (1999-2016)

- Patwardhan, B. et al. A critical analysis of the 'UGC-approved list of journals'. Curr. Sci. 2018;114: 1299-1303.

CHAPTER 2

Targeting Journals

When you have done your research work and plan a paper, you must target a suitable journal. As far as the timing is concerned, you should not wait to complete your entire research work for planning a paper.

Planning a paper:

When you are planning a paper, what should be the first step.

You will have to define it.

- What to publish (Content, extent, type): will deal with this later…
- Where to publish

Correlating what with where….

Correlating what you want to publish with where you want to publish is an essential aspect.

Major points targeting journal:

Some factors govern our decision to publish a paper in a journal. For deciding where to publish, we check three factors of a journal

- Impact

- Speed
- Reach

The Journal metrics answer these three factors. You need some checkpoints to know that this journal is suitable for you. And these three factors: impact, speed, and reach, decide the suitability of the journal for you.

Let us define "Journal Metrics."

"Journal metrics provide extra insight into three aspects of our journals – impact, speed and reach – and help authors select a journal when submitting an article for publication."
                                                                    - Elsevier

So "Impact speed and reach" are the key factors. Please do remember that you may have somewhat different targeting in your mind. Sometimes, you are ready to wait to publish in a good impact; sometimes, you are not ready to wait. So you will instead focus on a journal with good speed. And sometimes, you need to reach more and more people rather than focusing on impact and speed. Or sometimes the combination of these three aspects.

Impact means:

Let us discuss what does the impact means in academic writing? For example, you have written and published an article, and someone else built on your work and cites your article. That shows that your article impacted this, and in the same way, if lots of articles cite your work, it shows that your article had a significant impact. Now What the Bibliometrics (journal/ author metrics) does that shown impact can be expanded to the journal or researcher to prove their impact. From there, the impact can be spread even further. Your impact as a researcher spreads to a group like a faculty or the University. You can see that one cite from an article shows the impact on the entire linked system. This impact is not just the number, as some researchers feel. Their research is more than that. It is not like that a derivative work is trying to demolishing the previous work. A citation proves the IMPACT: an article has made an impact and becomes more important/useful. These bibliometrics are a more robust and useful tool in health/ biomedical and Sciences. Simultaneously, the other faculties like architecture, law, business, and engineering have the hurdles they need to cross. Engineering faculties tend to publish many harder to track conference papers and, therefore, more challenging to be cited. The arts' faculties love books, and the books have exact cites problems due to irregular publishing schedules making it harder to track. Law, on the other hand, has a different problem. However, they publish heavily in journals. Much of their work is aimed at judges and politicians rather than other academics. The architecture people have their unique problem because their lot of work has an artistic component that is hard to track and cite. The business has its problems. Mainly because bibliometrics is more focused on sciences, and these are just entering their domain now.

Speed

What does speed mean? Authors need to publish their work on time, especially in fast-moving research areas. Most of the time, early rejection is far better than very late acceptance. In the process of publication, the delay is more painful than rejection. In contrast, the journals that give rejection even in 48 hrs to one week are useful for communicating. The journals that clarify the authors about the suitability for further peer reviewing/ processing are well in time. It is not acceptable to remain in the dark or uncertain and plan the article for the new journal again without losing much more time.

See "The frequency of the journal": semiannual, quarterly, bimonthly, monthly, fortnightly, or weekly. You have to check the frequency of the journal for assessing the speed of publication. You can check two significant factors: "average number of weeks taken by the peer review process," "average number of weeks taken for first decision/final decision/ online/offline publication."

Reach

The third important factor is reach.

- Reach of journals to readers and authors: the popularity

- Wide geographical area: the global presence

- The number of downloads country-wise & The number of Corresponding author countrywide for the last 5 yr are the indicators of reach of the journal

Standards/metrics are needed:

- To assess the relative suitability of the journals

- To rank the journal on merit (Impact, Speed, Reach)

- To have the benchmark of competitiveness (we will be in a condition to decide the competitiveness only after seeing particular metrics) of journals

- To have the benchmark of competitiveness of authors: For assessing the researchers for a grant application, job/ promotion, awards etc.

- To attract more and more potential authors and the relevant research work

- To save time in targeting the most suitable journal by the authors, authors can not study several journals and spend their valuable time just choosing a suitable journal. The metrics save the researcher's time by helping him/her target the most suitable journal.

The metrics may be of two types Journal metrics and author metrics. Moreover, these may be further sub-classified, as shown in Table 1.

Table 1 Types of Metrics.

Journal metrics	**Author metrics**
• **IF**	• H index
• **ISI Ranking**	• I10 index
• **Citescore metrics**	• G index
• **Eigenfactor**	
• **Article Influence**	
• **Immediacy index**	
• **SNIP**	
• **SJR**	
• **Altmetrics**	
• **H5**	

Targeting Journal

For targeting your manuscript to a suitable journal, you must take care of the following points.

- Match your topic with the scope of journal

- Refer Databases for targeting

- Reputation (IF or other journal metrics: Impact, speed and reach)

- Time

- Availability (online/ offline)

- Indexing

- Format (See the guidelines for authors and general submission guidelines)

- APC

Match your topic with the scope of the journal:

Failing to match your topic with the journal's scope leads to rejection at the editorial level only, even before sending it to peer review.

Observe articles in the latest issue of Journal, Theme of issue or conference. Additional information required to decide are.

Refer Databases for targeting

You can refer the Literature databases like Endnote, Web of Science for searching a suitable journal. Enter you title, abstract and / or keywords, the database will give the list of suitable journal for your manuscript. Springer Author Academy also provide the opportunity for the authors to target the most suitable journal based on title and abstract. Apart from Springer's Journal suggester, Elsevier also provides a Journal finder for the authors. These are AI-based journal finders that provide much information like impact factor/ cite score, journal's speed, acceptance rate etc. You can decide as per your need.

Reputation (IF or other journal metrics: Impact, speed and reach)

Several ways can assess the reputation of a journal. Your own perception along with the opinion of your seniors (by their experience), type/quality of recent articles published in the journal, their importance, the presence of field experts in members of the Editorial Board, the acceptance rate of the journal and the journal's impact factor and other journal metrics may be the criteria of judging the reputation of a journal.

An author must overview these things before deciding to submit a paper to a particular Journal.

Time: Check how much time the journal takes for the peer-review process. This is very important to check the time taken by a journal in the review process. Target a journal that takes less time for the same. You cannot wait for years if you are planning an article with your Ph D thesis submission. In general, the minimum time is 2 to 3 months taken by a journal's review process.

Fast track processing of the article: If you can afford, avail it.

Availability (online/ offline):

The availability of the journal is also very important. Some journals are broadly available both online and in the print version. On the other hand, some journals are online-only or in print only. So, the article submission process may also be easy or complicated depends upon the journal's availability.

Indexing:

The journal indexing in the major electronic databases such as Medline, Biological Abstracts, Chemical Abstracts, or Current Contents must be checked before deciding to submit a paper to a journal.

Format (See the guidelines for authors and general submission guidelines):

Does the appearance of published articles – the format, typeface, and style used in citing references suite you as per your study or the research work? If relevant, does the journal publish short and/or rapid communications?

Article Processing/ Publishing Charges:

Apart from leading publishers' various open access journals, various print journals also bill the author for page charges, a cost per final printed page. Most journals have a separate charge for color plates. This may be as much as $1000 per color plate. Many journals will waive page charges if this presents a financial hardship for the author; color plate charges are less readily waived and would at least require evidence that the color is essential to the presentation of the data (e.g., to show a double-labelled cell).

In a nutshell, the quality journal should be targeted for publishing your manuscript. In general, the efforts should be focused to publish in journals with good impact (genuine impact factor); alternatively, the journals with good indexing like SCOPUS, Web of Science, SCI, ESCI and/or PubMed should be selected for publishing manuscript related to sciences, biomedical and pharmaceutical sciences.

Further Reading

- Selecting a Journal: https://youtu.be/XILmZp84Qf8
- https://utah.instructure.com/courses/306223/pages/picking-a-journal-for-the-manuscript
- https://www.springer.com/gp/authors-editors/journal-author/journal-author-academy
- How to Maximize Your Study's Visibility by Choosing the Right Journal, https://www.wiley.com/network/researchers/discover/how-to-maximize-your-studys-visibility-by-choosing-the-right-journal

- Find the right journal to publish your research, https://authorservices.wiley.com/author-resources/Journal-Authors/find-a-journal/index.html

References

- Fowler, J. (2011). Writing for professional publication. Part 8: Targeting the right journal. British Journal of Nursing (BJN), 20(4), 254.

- Henly, S. (2014). Finding the right journal to disseminate your research. Nursing Research, 63(6), 387.

- https://www.nirfindia.org/2018/Ranking2018.html

- https://www.timeshighereducation.com/

- The best universities in the world 2019, https://www.youtube.com/watch?v=9GNVbF140F8

- The Handbook of Academic Writing: A Fresh Approach By Rowena Murray; Sarah Moore Open University Press, 2006

- Introduction to Bibliometrics, UTS Library, https://www.youtube.com/watch?v=yBHneMkeUHA

- Faber J, Writing scientific manuscripts: most common mistakes, Dental Press J Orthod. 2017; 22(5): 113–117. doi: 10.1590/2177-6709.22.5.113-117.sar

- Ohwovoriole AE, Writing biomedical manuscripts part I: fundamentals and general rules.West Afr J Med. 2011 May-Jun;30(3):151-7.

- Ohwovoriole AE, West Afr J Med. Writing biomedical manuscripts part II: standard elements and common errors. 2011 Nov-Dec;30(6):389-99.

- https://www.nytimes.com/2014/06/19/science/researching-the-brain-of-writers.html

- Gwendolyn Bounds, How Handwriting Trains the Brain, Oct 5, 2010; https://www.wsj.com/articles/SB10001424052748704631504575531932754922518#articleTabes%3Darticle

- Nature News, Nature, 2018: doi: 10.1038/d41586-018-00927-4

- Nature News, Nature; 2016: doi:10.1038/nature.2016.19198

- Nature News, Nature; 2014: doi:10.1038/nature.2014.14684

- arxiv.org/abs/1707.01162 : Publish Or Impoverish: An investigation of the monetary reward system of science in China (1999-2016)

- Patwardhan, B. et al. A critical analysis of the 'UGC-approved list of journals'. Curr. Sci. 2018;114: 1299-1303.

CHAPTER 3

Impact Factor

Impact Factor (IF) is the most important basis of the selection of the journal. It is a measure of the reputation of a journal.

"Impact factor is a measure of the frequency with which the "average article" in a journal has been cited in a particular year."

A journal's Impact factor is presented by a digit followed by the year and name of IF providing agency in brackets. e.g. on the home page of Expert Opinion on Drug Delivery journal (http://www.tandfonline. com/toc/iedd20/current) 2019 Impact Factor: 4.838, Ranking: 32/270 Pharmacology & Pharmacy © 2020 Clarivate Analytics, 2020 release of the Journal Citation Reports®)

It's a dynamic index that changes based on citations and the number of papers every year.

Calculation of IF

"In any given year, the impact factor of a journal is the number of citations, received in that year, of articles published in that journal during the two preceding years, divided by the total number of articles published in that journal during the two preceding years." (https://en.wikipedia.org /wiki/Impact_factor)

For example, a journal's 2019 impact factor calculation will be:

IF (2019) = (Citations in yr 2019 from articles of yr 2018 + Citations in yr 2019 from articles of yr 2017)/(Published papers 2018 + Published papers 2017)

IF (2019) = (1450 + 1550) / (150 + 260) = 4.878

However, you need not to calculate these things yourself. These are the automated calculations and record which are kept/ tracked and given by several agencies.

And the next question is who these agencies are? Who does award IF to journals?

Impact Factor providing agencies

- Thomson Reuters/ Journal Citation Reports® (JCR®)/ Clarivate Analytics: If provided by JCR is mostly recognized across the subjects, countries and institutions.
- The Institute for Scientific Information ISI
- Scopus-SJR, CitesScore : a different set of the journal and author metrics is given by Scopus (will be discussed later).

Indexing Agencies

- Science Citation Index® (SCI®) and ESCI
- Social Sciences Citation Index® (SSCI®).
- PubMed: NCBI
- Web of Science
- SCOPUS
- EMBASE
- Chemical Abstracts
- ISI
- Index Copernicus
- Sci factor
- ICI
- Google Scholar (the most widespread coverage)

The higher the number of well-known indexing agencies by which the journal is indexed, the more potential the journal is for targeting the manuscript.

These indexing agencies index the journal articles, and once these journals are indexed in these indexing services, agencies like Clarivate keep track of the citations and publications and then provide IF from time to time. For example, JCR releases the IF in July. For example, in 2020 July, the IF of 2019 was released.

Note: self-declaration of IF by journals is not valid. These agencies are globally recognized for analyzing and releasing the IF. Self-declaration is giving the award to ourselves and is an unethical practice.

Factors affecting the Impact Factor

After going through the basics of IF, let us see the factors on which the IF is dependent:

- No. of papers published and citations: By definition, IF depend on both the number and citations directly.

- Presence in various Indexing services: More indexing, higher chances of citations and hence the IF

- Frequency of publication of journal: It is a very important factor. A journal published fortnightly publishes a greater number of papers and has good chances of higher citations compared to quarterly, bimonthly, and monthly journal. That's why the chances of getting more citations and improved IF are higher in these cases.

- Online nature and wide dissemination (OA): Being online is a prerequisite for getting IF. However, some journals are very prestigious but do not have IF. (especially in cases of arts and humanity journals). OA journals provide free full text and hence have more readership, higher chances of citation, and chances of getting IF.

- Publisher's policies of self-citation: Some journal poses conditions on authors to cite some the papers of their own journal/publisher, this increases their citations and hence the chances of improving IF

- Nature of journals (Review only/ Interdisciplinary): Review and interdisciplinary journals have wide coverage and readership. Review articles are almost always cited at a higher rate than that of a research paper with new data. Every article's introduction part almost always cite state of art and/or relevant review papers rather than describing the background in details. So, almost in every discipline, the review journals have higher IF. e.g. in Pharma sciences: ADDR, EODD. You check your field of research....

Miscellaneous factors: Manuscript/presentation/editorial quality:

- Manuscript Quality: Better the quality of the manuscript; more will be the citations.

- Presentation quality of manuscript makes it easy to follow by the readers and researchers. A nicely presented manuscript is likely to be cited more.

- Editorial quality: Many journals have started adding introductory video and data set with the manuscript as additional resources. This increases their presentation quality and reach. They put these article's intro video or abstract video onto social media like youtube/Facebook, resulting in more readership and hence the citations are expected to be increased.

Impact Factor in Academic Recognition

The Academic Performance Indicators (API) prescribed by the latest University Grants Commission of India for Career Advancement Scheme and are for assessing biodata of an academician for University Teaching jobs.

It allows 8 points for each research paper of a peer-reviewed/ UGC listed journal (for a single author)

This score for paper in the journal is augmented based on impact factor:

Paper in the refereed journal without impact factor – by 5 points

Paper with an impact factor less than 1 - by 10 points;

Papers with impact factor between 1 and 2 by 15 points;

Papers with impact factor between 2 and 5 by 20 points;

Papers with impact factor between 5 and 10 by 25 points;

Papers with an impact factor above 10 by 30 points.

Up to two authors 50 % each; more than two authors 70/30 (main, corresponding/ rest of the authors)

Therefore, the higher the impact factor of the journal you have published higher will be your API score.

The international agencies and universities also take the help of various journal metrics and author metrics to assess the performance and suitability. It may be the total IF of an author's publications, or it may be the number of citations or the number of SCI-indexed journal articles together with the citations. So, we can say that IF plays a vital role in assessing a researcher and faculty member's expertise and academic performance.

Therefore, please be careful and not fall into the trap of predatory journals that wrongly claim the high impact factor.

If you want to verify the journal's IF, either you should have the list of IF issued by the agencies or simply type the name of the journal in the google search bar; if it would have the actual IF, the google would show in the box otherwise not.... (However, it may not show you the current year's IF).

Other approaches

Search individual publisher's website like Bentham, Elsevier, Springer, chose the journal from their list and then open the Main page-- IF will be shown if exists with year and name of the agency.

But for other journals, Don't rely upon the IF shown in their home/main page; first, check whether the journal is indexed in SCI or ESCI by checking the SCI website. This measure is suitable for Science journals. But for Arts and humanities journals, SCI indexing and IF is very rare to find. These journals are not generally indexed by the indexing services dedicated to Sciences, biomedical etc. And in some cases, journals are not there in English, and if they exist, they are not online. So, In India, UGC constituted a committee Consortium for Academic and Research Ethics (CARE) to refine and strengthen research publication in all the disciplines. In the sciences, technology engineering, biomedical and allied subjects, the web of science and Scopus indexed journals have been excluded from the analysis. For the rest of the journals, the committee is given the task to analyze and list the approved journals, including the Social Sciences, arts, and humanities subjects.

So, you can have the idea that without IF or without any indexing, the journals need the analysis, certification or approval for considering them in API.

It's better to publish in high impact or journals indexed in good indexing agencies like SCOPUS/ Web of Science, SCI, ESCI, PubMed, EMBASE etc.

IF: Limitations

- "The IF is not perfect, but to be fair, every metric has its flaws."
- Just a single highly cited article can improve the IF of a journal.
- Being a Journal level metrics does not discriminate between good/lousy author/article.
- The worst article in a journal has the same IF as the best article in that same journal.
- IF is a slow process and does not always depict trues picture.
- The difference in frequency and subject of the journal does not allow meaningful comparison of a different subject's journals.
- Inclusion of self-citation

The Journal Impact Factor quartile

It is the quotient of a journal's rank in category (X) and the total number of journals in the category (Y), so that (X / Y) = Percentile Rank Z.

$$Q1: 0.0 < Z \leq 0.25$$
$$Q2: 0.25 < Z \leq 0.5$$
$$Q3: 0.5 < Z \leq 0.75$$
$$Q4: 0.75 < Z$$

Each subject category of journals is divided into four quartiles: Q1, Q2, Q3, Q4. Q1 is occupied by the top 25% of journals in the list; Q2 is occupied by journals in the 25 to 50% group; Q3 is occupied by journals in the 50 to 75% group, and Q4 is occupied by journals in the 75 to 100% group. Those who are publishing in Q1 journals are given more weightage than Q2, Q3 and Q4 of the same category. Therefore, even if your paper is published in a lower impact factor journal of Q1 compared to another person's article (of the same field) published in a higher impact factor journal of Quartile 4, the weightage of your paper is greater.

You can publish your work in good journals with impact factor even without paying even a single penny.

Alternatively, target journals with good indexing do not matter if currently, they are not having IF. Because these journals have the good chances of getting IF in near future. E.g. CDDT (PubMed and SCOPUS indexed journal without impact factor till 2017). It is very much possible that it gets IF this year only…

After discussing the Impact factor as the first and foremost journal metrics, let us discuss some more journal metrics.

5 Year Impact factor

The 5-Year IF extends the 2-year window of the regular IF. This normalizes the time frame limitation of the standard two-year calculation-based Impact Factor. It is suitable for slow-moving areas of research where the citation is slow and need more time.

"A base of five years may be more appropriate for journals in certain fields because the body of citations may not be large enough to make reasonable comparisons, or it may take longer than two years to publish and distribute, to lead to a longer period before others cite the work." - Elsevier

5 Yr IF (Year X) = ((Total No of articles cited for X-1,X-2,X-3,X-4 and X-5 Yr))/((Total number of published articles in X-1,X-2,X- 3,X-4 and X-5 years))

Pros and cons of this IF are more or less the same as that of regular IF. This gives the holistic approach and flexibility concerning time frame and some time the actual picture comes with 5Yr IF rather than the regular 2 Year IF. And you can see in most of the journals both the IF are generally mentioned in their Home Page of the journal.

CiteScore metrics, Eigenfactor, Article influence, SNIP, SJR, Altmetrics and H5 index are the other well-known journal metrics. But the impact factor is used most commonly for the sciences, life sciences, biomedical and pharmaceutical journal's benchmarking.

Further Reading

- Semalty A, Pedagogical Innovations and Research Methodology 2019 Module 40: Journal Metrics: Academic Writing, https://youtu.be/QeG8euhvDV0
- Semalty A, Academic Writing, SWAYAM MOOC, CC: Dr Ajay Semalty. https://swayam.gov.in

- Cross JO, Impact factors – The Basics, the e resource management Handbook, https://www.uksg.org/sites/uksg.org/files/19-Cross-H76M463XL884HK78.pdf
- The Impact of Impact Factors, http://www.springer.com/gp/partners/society-zone-issues/the-impact-of-impact-factors/4592
- Bergstrom CT and West J, Comparing Impact Factor and Scopus CiteScore, http://eigenfactor.org/projects/posts/citescore.php
- Scopus Tutorial: CiteScore metrics in Scopus, https://www.youtube.com/ watch?v=zOZ852yJ9bw
- SJR & SNIP versus IMPACT FACTOR, https://youtu.be/GGDB1y3SUyA
- https://www.metrics-toolkit.org/
- Altmetrics explained in under 2 minutes, https://www.youtube.com/watch?v=-E5BIf4h5DQ
- Measuring research impact, https://library.leeds.ac.uk/info/1406/research_support/17/measuring_research_impact

References

- Semalty Ajay, Journal Metrics I & II, SWAYAM MOOC, Academic Writing (www.swayam.gov.in)
- Impact factor, https://en.wikipedia.org/wiki/Impact_factor
- https://journalinsights.elsevier.com/journals/0888-613X/authors
- https://en.wikipedia.org/wiki/Impact_factor
- http://www.citefactor.org/journal-impact-factor-list-2014_I.html
- http://lms.uop.edu.jo/lms/mod/data/view.php?d=29&advanced=0&paging&page=1
- Research Indices - I: Impact Factor, https://www.youtube.com/watch?v=nPLnJqLEknY
- Introduction to Bibliometrics, UTS Library, https://www.youtube.com/watch?v=yBHneMkeUHA
- The EigenfactorTM metrics, December 2008The Journal of Neuroscience : The Official Journal of the Society for Neuroscience 28(45):11433-4, DOI: 10.1523/JNEUROSCI.0003-08.2008
- Crotty D, Journal Metrics, Article III; OtherMetrics: beyond the Impact Factor, Cardiopulse, doi:10.1093/eurheartj/ehx446
- Crotty D, Journal Metrics, Article IV; AltMetrics, Cardiopulse doi:10.1093/eurheartj/ehx447
- http://www.scopus.com

CHAPTER 4

Review Paper Writing

Reviews are the mirror of current status and the pathfinder for the future trends of a particular area of study. Reviews play an essential role in scientific communication and understanding. Well-written, critical reviews provide a necessary overview and integration of disparate fragments of rapidly advancing knowledge in a speciality or subspecialty. As such, they can elucidate trends in research and point to unanswered questions that provide opportunities for future study. Reviews also give science policymakers as well as researchers a clearer insight into the potential importance of emerging knowledge.

Defining Review Papers

"Review papers are systematically organized compilation of a specific body of knowledge which aims to critically study, summarize and synthesize the author's opinion or highlight the development of the field with time."

A review paper does not describe the author's own work generally but rather synthesizes ideas and results from other research papers that have been published in a certain subject area. However, analytical or critical reviews may have some of the author's work. Generally, a person who has experience of research on a particular area of study should only be expected to write a review. A review is not just a compilation of studies. It is the analytical or critical view of the study area, i.e. strength, weakness, opportunity, and threats (SWOT analysis).

This requires a different sort of research: a complete review of this literature in the chosen area. Moreover, a good research paper is more than a descriptive "listing" of various scientific studies' findings, like a glorified annotated bibliography. Instead, this paper should be a thoughtful integration of the results and ideas coming from a number of studies to provide a new perspective or understanding or provoke discussion within that field. The conclusions of several studies need to be placed in perspective with one another... do they agree? If not, how might the apparent conflicts be solved? What might be productive areas to research in the future? A useful resource for a student writing a review paper is the "Annual Reviews", which are available for a number of fields. Section II of this book provides a large number of pharmaceutical journals specially dedicated to reviews. Almost each research journal publishes a few quality reviews in each of its issues.

But the review writing practice is not promoted and encouraged as that of research articles among researchers. One reason is that writing reviews are a uniquely demanding and intensive task. There was a time when tracking down relevant references to a subject in libraries was a major undertaking. That alone discouraged many scientists from writing reviews. While the situation today isn't perfect, it has improved significantly. The wealth of information sources available on the Internet, online databases, and document-delivery services makes locating and retrieving basic information on most topics, both feasible and affordable.

Another reason a scientist avoids writing reviews is the lack of professional recognition. Promotion and tenure committees still tend to place the highest value on original research articles, and reviews are not given equal weight. Funding agencies probably share this bias against reviews in their decision making. Even scientists may be guilty of exalting original research articles over other types of publications, although reviews are more frequently cited. But most of the scientists, if asked to list their most significant publications-as many tenures and granting agencies often request-include reviews among their top five or ten contributions.

Importance of writing reviews

The review papers writing is required for one or more following purposes.

- To provide a ready reference for students
- To provide a ready reference for new researchers
- To develop an understanding of the knowledge domain
- To integrate rapidly advancing knowledge
- To elucidate trends in research and to point out the research gaps
- To help in origin and incubation of idea of research
- To improve the "h" index of authors
- To provide help in policymaking

Major aspects of a review paper

As discussed earlier, a review paper is all about the following aspects.

- It is always a uniquely demanding and intensive task.
- It is all about summarizing and synthesizing ideas
- It is expected to be written by experts if the research field.
- It requires a focused approach to present all the related aspects.
- It must be complete in all sense in covering the specific topic covered.
- It must be able to provide a critical presentation of the current status of the field of study and also be able to trigger future research.

Planning Review paper

Writing a review paper should be started in the later stage of planning your research topic itself. At the literature review stage, where you identify the problem and outline the tentative aim and objective review, writing can be started. And the writing process can be done along with the continuing literature review.

If you are not doing research, no time constraint is there; just start after doing a proper literature review on the desired topic. Faculty members can also plan reviews from their academic experience. It may serve as an advanced compilation or overview. Advanced lecture-note style reviews are desired by some journals/ thematic issues.

Major Considerations in Review Writing

- Try to make your research paper an integrated synthesis of the literature rather than a jumbled regurgitation of facts. It will ease the designing and writing of the review on the topic.

- Give enough time in literature review and planning a review paper. For a 10-20 page paper, it ideally takes a month to carry out the library searches and to collect the necessary materials.

- Start out with a clear idea of the question you are trying to answer in the paper. Write it somewhere and show it to an advisor to see if it makes sense, is "do-able", etc. In general, a simple, specific idea is easier to research and to write about. Equally, it must be interesting and inclusive enough to ensure there's enough material available to review.

- Do the exhaustive literature review. Make sure you are familiar with all the resources available to help you locate references.

- Take notes, including full citations (authors' names, journal, date and page number) from each paper as you read it. Use index cards or a word processor. Index cards are nice in that you can shuffle them around, color code ideas on them, highlight etc. The advantage of using a word processor is that you will later be able to use your notes to cut and paste together the first draft, plus you'll have all your citations there already, which saves time when building your citation list. Organize your notes. "Where <u>did</u> I read that?" is the plague of all writers. The better organized your notes; the less this is a problem.

- Outline your paper before doing anything else! This will help you to organize your thoughts and will markedly improve the overall quality of your final product. Discuss with your supervisor/ team members/ coauthors. Also, discuss and plan what type of review you want to write?

- Try to be specific and focused while pinpointing your objective and targeting a topic. This will help you organise the literature review (LR) and your thoughts and improve your paper's quality. The review is not always the complete LR you have performed. Do not copy-paste your LR in a review paper. It is just a specific section of the LR. It has got a different approach.

- Don't be afraid to write your ideas down before they are perfectly formed. If you can get them down on paper, you can place them in a logical sequence and develop them into a flowing presentation later.

- Use the draft system: Write a first draft. Leave it for a day or two. Come back to it and revise it as much as you can, then let someone read it. Once they have read it, revise the paper again. Respond to your reviewer's comments and also clarify any passages that seemed to confuse them. Expect that your paper will need revisions, and don't feel bad when that turns out to be true.

- Don't write in the first person (I think). This reduces your credibility. Write with authority (It is, they do)

Targeting journal for review Paper

In the previous chapter, we have already dealt with the aspect of targeting journal for papers. For review papers, the following points must be considered for targeting journals.

- Match your objectives and expectations
- Match your topic with the scope of journal
- Check the Journal metrics based on your choice related to impact, speed and reach.
- Check the Article Processing/Publishing Charges (APC)
- Check the level of Review Articles in the Target Journal
- Match with the Author's Guidelines

These are the major factors of targeting a journal. Enlist your expectation and match them with journal's aura. If it matches, then only target the journal. Moreover, the fresh researchers should not target very high impact journals (like Advanced Drug Delivery Reviews, Nature, Expert Opinion on Drug Delivery etc.) for the early publications as review papers.

Designing and Writing a review paper

When writing a review paper, your job is to present what is known about a specific topic and to synthesize all the unconnected threads of the individual studies into an integrated "State of the Science" type of review. In your paper, you will outline the overall picture of your topic area; scientists in that field currently understand it. Your paper should clearly outline any problems currently being addressed and explain the basis of any conflicts between experts in the field. If there are important conflicts as a reviewer, you are in a position to suggest which side of the conflict has the weight of evidence supporting it and why. For conflicts that, in your opinion, do not yet have a clear resolution, you are also in a position to makes suggestions as to the types of experiments that need to be done to resolve those arguments.

Your review paper should have the following sections:

(a) **Title:** Like a research paper, this should be short and inform your reader of the major ideas that will be discussed. Preferably plan 4-5 titles in the planning stage, but finalize it at last.

(b) **Abstract:** Again, this should be written last and should summarize the major points made within the body of your paper.

(c) **Introduction:** Your introduction should be short and concise. It should not have separate headings from the body of the paper. The purpose of the introduction is to introduce your reader to the ideas that you will be addressing in the body of your paper. In your introduction, you should be trying to bring readers from different backgrounds up to speed with the "thesis" or objective of your paper and explain to them why it is that this issue is important. It is not a review of the field... that is what the body of the paper is for! It is generally written after the body of the paper is completed (so that you know where you've "gone" intellectually in the paper and thus can effectively communicate to your reader what to expect). Therefore, the Introduction section of a review paper gives the importance of the topic, seeks the reader's attention, creates interest, and tells a story.

(d) **Body:** In this portion of your paper, you will outline the background for your idea and begin to synthesize ideas from the papers you've read in order to build a coherent "thesis". Before you write this section, figure out what your perspective is going to be (what are you trying to show?). Having done this, try to present your ideas in such a way that they build your discussion logically towards your goal. Outlines will be a big help to you at this stage. Frequently using headings (e.g. History of the idea, Specific conflicts, etc.) can help you systematically address each important point that you wish to make and help your reader follow your arguments. Once you've developed your headings, you can then go back and place topic sentences for each paragraph of information you wish to convey under the appropriate heading. Each paragraph should have clear, well thought out points and should contain only the information needed to make or support that point. Fill in each paragraph with more details until you have a coherent argument building towards your final, concluding statement. The review paper should have the quality infographics (figure/ table etc.) in an optimum number.

(e) Conclusion: As the introduction, the conclusion section is not usually separated from the body of the paper, although it can be if it is really long. In this section, you should restate your paper's objective(s) and point out how you have satisfied these goals. It should also reiterate what the major conclusions (ideas) of your study are.

(f) Acknowledgements: Again, this should include only people who made considerable impact on your research... people with whom you had fruitful discussions, a librarian who spent hours with you trying to track down an elusive publication that was key to your research etc.

(g) Literature Cited. Should follow the standard format outlined by the journal in which you will publish.

After writing the first draft, leave it for some days (but not weeks). Keep thinking. Come back to it and revise it as much as you can. Give it to someone to read. And seek advice and inputs. Revise the paper again. Identify what and where is the gap in the story you are trying to tell. Keep on noting down references for citation (Literature management). Consult with your team/ supervisor, brainstorm. It cannot be said precisely how many times it needs revision. It depends on your LR, subject and level.

Keep on formatting the article as per the author's instructions. Follow the writing style recommended by the journal. Stick to the guidelines of the journal. You can avoid rejection by following the guidelines also.

Once the article is ready, along with all the related figure and table, submit it to the targeted journal at the earliest. Delaying submission of a review paper may demand the updating of the same again. The review comments must be addressed assertively, humbly and professionally. You must include/exclude/modify the content of the manuscript, as suggested by reviewers.

Special care must be taken to proofread the final version of the article sent after the paper's acceptance. Check for any page break, missing content/table/figure or the misplacement of table or figures. Sometimes the graphical or video abstract are also demanded by some journals at the final stage. Do plan an effective infographic as a graphical abstract.

Points to Remember

- Once you have prepared a final draft and revised the review, send the manuscript ASAP for publication.

- Always cover the topic fully with a focus and make a chronological rhythm.

- Include the latest references as much as possible (in tune with the journal targeted) to give the idea of the current trend of the topic.

- Never include unpublished results of studies relevant to the topic.

- Try to be unique and focused on the presentation of the topic.

Further Reading

- Guidance of a review paper, https://www.journals.elsevier.com/ international-journal-of-machine-tools-and-manufacture/news/ guidance-for-review-papers

- Literature review paper, http://websites.uwlax.edu/biology/Review Papers.html

- https://www.springer.com/gp/authors-editors/journal-author/journal-author-academy/15186

- Fundamentals of manuscript preparations, https://researcher academy.elsevier.com/writing-research/fundamentals-manuscript-preparation

References

- Anson, Chris M. and Robert A. Schwegler. The Longman Handbook for Writers and Readers. 6th edition. New York: Longman, 2010.

- Types of reviews, http://library.atmiya.net/research%20commons/research guide/literature_review.php

CHAPTER 5

Writing a Research Paper

A research paper writing has the following crucial and equally important components.

1. Planning
2. Writing
3. Editing & Revising
4. Submitting Manuscript & Follow-ups
5. Avoiding Rejection

The sections ahead shall be focused on all the above components of research paper writing.

1. Planning

As we plan the research work carefully the same holds true for the research paper. A complete and thorough planning of various aspects of research paper increases the chance of its publication. An author must plan many a thing before beginning of writing a scientific paper. Some general important aspects are discussed as followed.

Type of paper: As far as the planning of paper is concerned the first step is to decide at the onset, whether it should be presented as a review article, original article, short communication, or letter to the editor.

Target the journal: According to the concerned field of study, the journal to which paper is to be communicated should be selected carefully. The target readers should also be decided in advance for the paper. The paper must be written with the target audience or readers in mind and to an appropriate Journal that is read by that audience. Therefore, it is very important to finalize the journal to which the paper be communicated at the outset. There are several factors to consider when choosing a journal. It is unlikely that one journal will have all the features you are looking for, so you may have to compromise. However, there is one essential feature that you should not compromise on – *manuscripts must be peer reviewed for publication if they are to be considered as research articles.*

What type of research does the journal publish? Is its focus broad or narrow? Which disciplines are represented? What is the journal's orientation – for example, is it clinical or basic, theoretical, or applied?

Language: English is the most widespread language with respect to readership in international scientific communication. Thus, if you are interested in communicating your results widely to the international scientific community, then it is essential to publish in English. If, on the other hand, you wish to communicate to a more localized community (e.g., physicians in a particular geographical area), you might choose a journal that permits another language. Some journals which are published in other languages (e.g., Swiss journals) also allow submission and publication in English along with the other official language of the journal.

Indexing: The journal indexing in the major electronic databases such as Medline, Biological Abstracts, Chemical Abstracts, or Current Contents must be checked before deciding to submit a paper to a journal.

Availability: The availability of the journal is also very important. Some journals are broadly available both online and in print version. On the other hand, some journals are online only or in print only. So, the article submission process may also be easier or the complex depending upon the availability of the journal.

Reputation: The reputation of a journal can be assessed by several ways. Your own perception along with the opinion of your seniors (by their experience), type/quality of recent articles published in the journal, their importance, the presence of field experts in members of the Editorial Board, the acceptance rate of the journal and the journal's *impact factor* may be the criteria of judging the reputation of a journal. An author must overview these things before deciding to submit a paper to journal.

Impact Factor: The journal impact factor is a measure of the frequency with which the "average article" in a journal has been cited in a particular year. The impact factor will help you evaluate a journal's relative importance, especially when you compare it to others in the same field. The impact factor is calculated by dividing the number of current citations to articles published in the two previous years by the total number of articles published in that period. We have discussed the importance of Impact factor in previous chapter.

Immediacy Index: The journal Immediacy Index is a measure of how quickly the "average article" in a journal is cited. The Immediacy Index will tell you how often articles published in a journal are cited within the same year. The Immediacy Index is calculated by dividing the number of citations to articles published each year by the number of articles published in that year. The Immediacy Index is useful in comparing how quickly journals are cited. For comparing journals specializing in cutting-edge research, the Immediacy Index can provide a useful perspective.

Format: Does the appearance of published articles – the format, typeface, and style used in citing references suite you as per your study or the research work? If relevant, does the journal publish short and/or rapid communications?

Figures: The figures published in the journal have the resolution that you need or not? Color figures are charged or free?

Time to Print: The time taken by a journal from the receipt of the article to its publication is indicative of the time taken by the review process. So as per your need you can select a good journal with fast review process.

Charges: Apart from the various open access journals of leading publishers, various print journals also bill the author for *page charges*, a cost per final printed page. Most journals have a separate *charge for color plates*. This may be as much as $1000 per color plate. Many journals will waive page charges if this presents a financial hardship for the author; color plate charges are less readily waived and would at least require evidence that the color is essential to the presentation of the data (e.g., to show a double-labeled cell).

The targeting of journal decision must be taken early so that starting from the first draft, the paper may be written in the style and format of the Journal. Once you decide on a journal, obtain, and read that journal's *Instructions to Authors.* This document describes the format for your article and provides information on how to submit your manuscript. You can usually obtain a copy of the journals' Instructions to Authors on their website or in the first issue of a new volume.

Its good to go for monthly peer reviewed journals in beginning and when you get a few publications you can go for the international journals having high impact factor. Though we feel that if your article is rejected by a reputed journal it provides you a lot of valuable feedback for improving your writing skill. The reviewer's comments may help you to get back to a new journal with higher chances of acceptance. So, even the rejection from a reputed journal is a nice learning process without paying even a single penny.

Planning of Author's Name: At this stage itself, it is better to decide on the authorship. The definition of who should be an author (and in what order the list should be provided) varies with the field, the culture, and even the research group. Because of this potential for ambiguity, the rules to be used for determining authorship, including the order of authors, should be clearly agreed upon at the outset of a research work.

In academic research work the first author and the principal/ corresponding author gets more credit than the other co-authors. The point-based credit system (prescribed by University Grants Commission, Govt. of India) for assessing the research work and biodata of an academician for University jobs allows 8 points for each research paper of a peer reviewed and indexed journal. If there are more than one author of Research paper the points will be shared as follows:

- Up to three authors: Points will be shared equally,
- More than three authors; the first/Principal author and the corresponding author/ supervisor/ mentor of the teacher would share equally 70% of the total points and the remaining 30% would be shared equally.

Our belief is that authorship denotes an "intellectual contribution" to the work, and that an author should be able to explain and defend the work. This definition of authorship is probably the most common one among researchers and journal editors. Note that within this framework, "honorary authorship" - listing someone as an author who has **not** made an intellectual contribution (e.g., the head of the department or that individual who provided the funds)- would be considered unethical. See the Journals guidelines for knowing the presentation of author detail like name and affiliation.

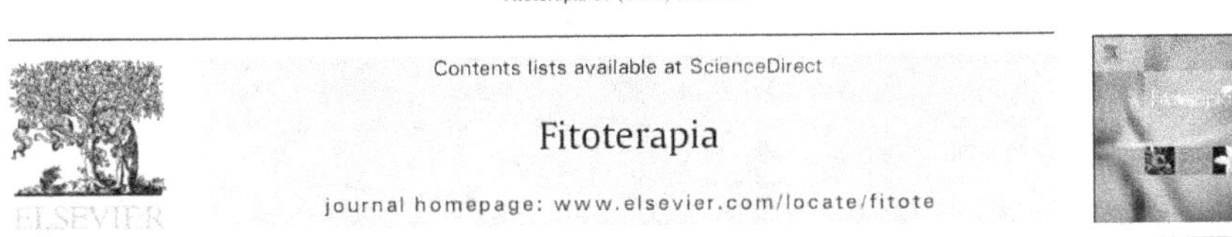

Fig. 1. Author's names presentation from different affiliations.

As you can see in this example of one of our paper of Fitoterapia, the full names are there. The first & last name are separated by the comma and the affiliations are marked with a and b and given after their names alternatively (Fig. 1).

In another title, it is a paper of our team from Indian drugs journal (Fig. 2). In this, last name is followed by the initials of the first name, separated by comma. So, it depends on the journal's guidelines on how the name should be mentioned in author details.

Independent of the method used to determine authorship, it is essential that all authors have given their consent to be designated as such and have approved the final version of the manuscript. One author is chosen as the "corresponding author." The editor of the journal will direct all correspondence to this individual who then has responsibility for keeping the other authors up to date regarding the status of the manuscript.

REVIEW ARTICLE

HERBAL HAIR GROWTH PROMOTION STRATEGIES FOR ALOPECIA

Semalty M.*, Semalty A., Joshi G.P. and Rawat M.S.M.

(Received 21 May 2008) (Accepted 30 July 2008)

ABSTRACT

Hairs are considered to be a major component of an individual's general appearance. Hair loss creates the psychosocial impact and results in a measurably detrimental change in self-esteem. Extensive researches are going on to explore the effective and safe drug for hair growth. Angiogenesis (through endogenous substances), androgen antagonism, potassium channel opening and 5-alpha reductase inhibition are the major non-surgical therapeutic strategies of hair growth promotion. Only two drugs minoxidil and finasteride have been approved by US FDA for hair growth promotion. Herbal drugs are also being investigated for potential and safer alternatives. The article focuses on causes and factors affecting hair loss. The developments in hair rejuvenation strategies are discussed along with the potential of herbal drugs for hair growth activity.

Fig. 2. Author's names presentation: Indian Drugs (SCOPUS indexed journal).

Planning the studies to be included: The most relevant and new studies should be incorporated to clear the current development in the topic with respect to the background of the research work. And this planning should be made with great attention and accuracy. Studies included must be related in a sense to reach to a solid conclusion.

The review articles should not only cover the topic in totality but also should discuss the topic with a critical overview. So, the articles included must be selected in such a way that it critically explains the objective.

Observing

Once the Journal is finalized the next step in designing a paper is observing various aspects of the journal which may guide the writing of paper. The following elements of the journal are needed to be observed.

Articles in latest issue of journal: Observe the articles published in the latest issue of the targeted journal. Observe the writing styles, titles, formatting styles, soundness of contents of the articles, presentation of results and discussion. Also observe whether the online submission of manuscript is allowed or not.

Theme of issue or conference: If a journal publishes theme-based issues, then the title of the paper must match the theme of the issue. In caser of sending papers for a conference, observe the theme of the conference and try to send the paper of same or most related topic. These will enhance the probability of acceptance of the paper.

Additional information required: Observe what additional information and certificates are asked by the publisher of journal. Get the appropriate ethical, statistical, and copyright clearance for the paper in the beginning itself. It is always better to collect and prepare illustrations, tables, graphs, and photographs before you start out.

2. Writing

The very first thing to keep in your mind is that to write a paper is neither too easy nor too tough. Some additional points to ponder over are:

1. Provide utility-based research article with systematic and complete presentation.
2. Be honest in presenting the data and the text.
3. Write in simple and clear scientific English.
4. Neither copy the work nor split the work in various research papers.

Paper must be written in clear and simple writing style with the vital incorporation of original and good scientific data. Before start writing determine the basic format of the article.

Time to Start writing

You must start the writing, before finishing your entire experimental work. Writing often triggers new ideas: you may realize that there are additional experiments to run or additional parameters that you need to add. If you wait until you are done in the lab, have dismantled the equipment, and possibly moved on to another position, you will not have the opportunity to test these ideas.

Time to publish

It is time to publish when your findings represent a complete story (or at least a complete chapter), one that will make a significant contribution to the scientific literature. Simply collecting a given amount of data is not adequate.

Determine the basic format

There are three basic formats for peer-reviewed research articles:

Full-length research articles: These articles contain a comprehensive investigation of the subject matter and are viewed as the standard format. It uses the "IMRAD" format – Introduction, Methods, Results, and Discussion.

Short (or brief) communications: While not as comprehensive in scope as full-length research articles, these papers also make a significant contribution to the literature. Their length will be set by the journal but is usually 3500 words or less and will contain up to 1-2 tables and figures. Unlike full papers, methods, results, and discussions may be combined into a single section.

Rapid communications: These articles quickly disseminate particularly "hot" findings, usually in a brief communication format. Firstly, a rough draft of the paper is prepared. At this stage one should plan the architecture or the basic structure which comprises of the sections which appear in a journal style paper in the following prescribed order:

Experimental process	Section of Paper
What did I do in a nutshell?	Abstract
What is the problem?	Introduction
How did I solve the problem?	Materials and Methods
What did I find out?	Results
What does it mean?	Discussion
Who helped me out?	Acknowledgments (optional)
Whose work did I refer to?	References
Extra Information	Tables & Figures

Besides this basic body of the text of the paper, there is one important and vital element the *title*. In the following sections we shall discuss each component of a research paper.

Title

This is the reader's first encounter with the paper in the content page of a Journal. The title will decide whether the reader will turn to that page of the Journal and would want to read on. The title must, therefore, be descriptive. It must also be short and simple worded to catch the reader's attention. Although attractive titles are more eye catching, they should avoid sensationalism. A good, reliable, and simple technique is to briefly write the question that was asked, or the answer that was arrived at the end of the study.

Abstract

Initially before start of the study, writing out an abstract is like the trailer of a film, and this is about as far as most readers will go while scanning a Journal. A good abstract provides 150-250 words of all the information about the paper; the aim of the study, the methodology used, the results obtained, and the conclusions drawn. A good abstract stands alone. Most Journals demand a structured abstract where the abstract is split into subheadings objectives, methods, results, and conclusions.

Considerable time must be spent in writing the abstract since the editor will usually make up his mind about accepting or rejecting the paper by merely reading the abstract.

Introduction

When writing an introduction, remember that you are not narrating a story, and neither is the 'introduction' a review of the subject. It should be mentioned clearly "what do you want to do" and "why you did it". In other words, spell out the question or hypothesis that your research aimed to settle. Also explain why the research was undertaken, were there gaps in the existing knowledge or was any existing data conflicting in its conclusions and therefore the present study. Start with the brief background and brief literature review, introduce the topic, identify research gap, define problem, present rationality and novelty, and then present your way out what you did in the study.

The last para of the introduction must address your hypothesis leading to aim & objective and methods of the present form. Be concise, develop the cohesion and coherence in the entire introduction, follow the logical transition. Remember the reader is an expert, write for him not for a layman.

Materials and Methods

The difference of this section in comparison to the thesis or post-graduation (M. Pharm./ M. Tech.) dissertation is the length of the section. Discuss the methodology logically and in a concise way. In the materials give the materials used and other sources, subject chosen, Area of research etc in case of field Study. In the research paper well established or previously methods are not reported. They just can be cited.

Have clarity in reporting methods. It is important because it is the point which makes your work reproducible and reproducibility is the key feature of any research article. A reader should be able to reproduce your research by following your methods. So, it must be clear.

Instrument software name, model, version, company etc must be mentioned wherever used. Statistical method and level of significance/ acceptance criteria must be mentioned clearly. Necessary permissions should be included like ethical committee approvals, herbarium numbers. You must include or if you are following a particular protocol from an official guideline, you must mention that.

In material and methods, you can also include the figures like a flowchart of a process for easy understanding, the image of subject study area, plant map etc. You can add as an image but remember the image must be plagiarism free.

As far as the tense is concerned you must write this section in the past tense or past perfect tense. And in most cases, it is in the past tense.

Results & Discussion

In the section, try to answer what was the outcome of problem treatment from a hypothesis. It must be evidence-based. This section provides evidence that leads to the answers of the study to the question you post at the start. The presentation must be professional. State the results without any bias. Do not exaggerate the results. Do not be afraid of reporting negative results. So, even if some paradox is there, some contradicting results are there, report them also. Statistical support must be mentioned. Use good statistics to show the result. In the modern era, there is no research article which is accepted, and which is not having statistical tools or use of suitable statistical tools to show the significance of the results. Equation and special characters must be given due attention. The presentation of the equation must be given due attention. It is better to write the equations in Microsoft equation. Here again, you will write it in the past tense or past perfect tense, and the last feature is completeness. Cover all the parameters. You must cover all the parameters, and the results must be complete.

In the discussion, try to answer how was the outcome of problem treatment correlated and or contradicted with the previous studies?

Take the result one by one and discuss them. Discuss the results, considering existing knowledge. Be critical, discuss the results with clarity and reader friendliness and use the references freely to support discussion.

Acknowledgments (included as needed)

The purpose of this section is to recognize and thank those individuals and organizations whose contributions to the work presented should be acknowledged but are not extensive enough to merit authorship.

When applicable, the following information is presented in this order:

1. Individuals (or Organization) other than authors who made a significant contribution to the research by donating important reagents or materials, collecting data, providing extensive advice on drafts of the manuscript, etc. Typically, the nature of the contribution is noted, for example

   The authors thank to Dr Reddy's Lab for providing the gift sample of diltiazem hydrochloride.

2. If the work has been presented at a conference, then this is often noted. For example,

   Portions of this work were presented at the 25th Annual Conference of IPA Meeting, December 1-3, 2005, Hydearbad, INDIA.

3. Organizations that funded the research or provided free analytical or other services must be acknowledged. The general format for this information is

   The authors thank grant provided by the UGC, New Delhi (37-643/2009) for the research work.

Note that it is ***essential*** to get permission from any individual whose help is acknowledged. Also, many scientific societies and journals are indicating that it is essential to disclose any financial support that has been provided for the work.

References

The purpose of this section is to provide the full citation for article referenced in the text.

A complete reference includes all the authors' names, the title of the article, the journal name, the volume number, page numbers, and the year of publication. A wide range of styles is used for citing references in the text and bibliography. Check the journal's *Instructions to Authors* for information about the content and formatting of references.

Within the text, articles are cited by providing the author and year of the article (e.g., Nagai and Junginger, 1996). When there are more than two authors, the first author is provided together with *e. al.* (e.g., Fischer et al..., 1996). If more than one reference is cited for a given point, they are usually listed in chronological order (e.g., Nagai and Junginger, 1995; Junginger et al., 1996). If there is any ambiguity, a letter can be added to the year of publication (e.g., Junginger et al., 1995a; 1995b).

At the end of the paper a list of references, or bibliography, is provided. This list must be limited to the references cited within the text and most often is provided in alphabetical order.

In some cases, citations appear in the text as numbers, usually a superscript, which then refer to a particular item in the reference list.

It is the obligation of the authors to provide a scholarly listing of the primary references of relevance to the paper. Authors are obliged to do a thorough review of the key areas of the scientific literature as part this process. In general, original *research* articles rather than *review* articles should be cited, and the research articles should be the earliest ones that made the finding.

It is essential that authors check each reference that they cite. Simply copying a reference from the bibliography of a published paper is inadequate since errors in referencing are very common. In checking a reference, authors must not only make sure that the citation is accurate but also that the text supports the point for which it being used as a reference. The reference checking and validation facility is provided by various free web-based service providers. The reference is validated through their unique digital object identifier (Doi) identity number or PUBMED i.d. number. Doi-numbers and PUBMED i.d. can be easily assigned by using the free web-service at   http://www.crossref.org/SimpleTextQuery   (just   copy   your reference list into the box and press 'submit'). Many a times, when you submit a paper online to an international journal, the manuscript handling website provide you the opportunity to see the validation report of your references. This allows and encourages the use of most accessible references only. Some time your article may get rejected just based on validation report of references. Say for example, in the research article submitted by you, if out of 30 references used in the article, 15 to 20 are not validated (i.e., with no doi number and PubMed id), then your article may be summarily rejected without being referred to reviewers by the editor himself. The aim of validation of references is to provide the easily accessible references to the reviewers and readers of the article.

References that are not readily available or are in a language not understood by the author present a particular challenge. In the former case, most libraries provide a service that enables authors to obtain papers from a wide range of other libraries. An alternative that is sometimes available is to directly contact the author of the article in question and request a copy.

Articles in foreign languages sometimes provide enough information in their tables and figures to permit an accurate comprehension of their results, even if the language itself is not understood. In this regard it is helpful that several scientific terms are the same in English as in many other languages. Alternatively, it usually is possible to have an article translated by a local service.

If a reference cannot be checked by the author, the only alternative to not citing it is to cite it as a secondary reference (e.g., Hooke, 1665, as cited in Fischer, 1995).

If citations are needed for more than one point in a sentence, it is helpful for the reader if the citations appear throughout the sentence, rather than as a collection at the end. For example,

Previous studies have shown that this compound can exist in a solid (Wang and Beauford, 1993), liquid (Jones et al., 1992), or gaseous (Diaz, 1995) state.

Length: Ideally, a paper will list all the references necessary to document each point that is made by the authors. In practical terms, however, most journals will impose a limit to conserve space. A rule of thumb is no more than 6 references for a particular point and no more than 100 references per paper.

Tables and Figures

The purpose of this section is to report data that are too numerous or complicated to be described adequately in the text; to reveal trends or patterns in the data.

It contains tables; possible figures include graphs (bar, line, scatter), diagrams, cartoons (i.e., chemical structures or mechanisms), and photographs. Figures are usually in black and white. Color is extremely expensive to publish and should only be used when it provides unique information.

Number: Limit the number of tables and figures to those that provide essential information that could not adequately be presented in text.

Table and Figure Legends

The purpose of this section is to provide a knowledgeable reader with the information required for understanding the table or figure.

The composition of a legend depends on the item it refers to. It should provide information regarding the conditions of the experiment, but not give a summary or interpretation of the results. In addition, statistical information is often provided. This may include

1. The number of times an experiment was performed, or a condition was tested.
2. What the values in the table or figure represent, for example *mean, S.E.M.* (standard error of the mean)
3. The statistical test used in analyzing the data
4. Whether the test was "one-tailed" or "two-tailed" (if relevant)
5. The *p* value that was used in determining significance
6. If an asterisk or other mark is used in the table or graph to denote statistically significant results, then this mark should be defined.

For example, the statistics portion of a figure legend might look like this,

*n=5 for each condition. Values represent mean $\pm$ S.E.M. Data were analyzed using a one-tailed Student's t-test. * denotes significance, p < 0.05.*

Tense: Past tense.

Style: Each table and figure should be understandable on its own, without reference to the text.

Within a manuscript, the placement of the legend varies depending on whether it refers to a table or figure:

Table: The title, table, and legend should appear on the same page, in the order listed.

Figure: Each figure should appear on a separate page. The numbered legends are listed one after another (i.e., several to a page). The title for a figure comprises the first sentence in the figure legend.

3. Editing & Revising

This step involves three major tasks, each to be carried out in the order given:

1. *Make major alterations*: Fill in gaps, correct flaws in logic, restructure the document to present the material in the most logical order.

2. *Polish the style*: Refine the text, then correct grammar and spelling.

3. *Format the document:* Make your manuscript attractive and easy to read

It is important to do the tasks in the stated order. Otherwise, you may find yourself spending a lot of time revising material that you later delete.

Self-Revision by the Author(s)

Revision of your writing is an on-going process from the time you begin until the final copy is submitted. A strategy that works for many people is to write out an initial draft in total without substantial revision and then let it sit for a day. Come back to it then and begin revising your paper as per the following perspectives and orders.

- check the sequence of ideas/background/content in each section for logical progression (*your topic sentences should do this*).

- check for a strong relationship of ideas between the Introduction (*what we knew before our study*) and the Discussion (*how our study changes or supports our previous understanding*).

- check that each paragraph has a **coherent topic sentence**, most often as the lead sentence.

- in each paragraph do the **other sentences support the topic sentence**.

- check the **transitions between paragraphs** to ensure they are *logical* and *smooth*.

- check for *consistent* and *correct* use of **terminology.**

- can you change a passive verb construction to an **active verb**?

- eliminate **superfluous lead phrases** (*Once that was done, ..*).

- remove all **colloquial language.**

- check for **redundancy** (i.e., places where you repeat what you have said elsewhere).

- read each sentence closely for **clarity** and **brevity. Can you say the same thing with fewer words?**

- **Read the paper aloud** to find those quirky sentences that you wrote while still half asleep - if does not sound correct when spoken aloud, it will read even more oddly.

- **Be sure to use spell check.** It will help you catch most typos and many wrongly spelled words. But do not let it replace anything automatically, or you will end up with nonsense words. You will still have to read through your piece and use a print dictionary or writer's handbook to look up words that you suspect are not right.

- **Do not depend on a thesaurus and grammar checker**. The best ones still miss many errors, and they give a lot of bad advice. If you know that you overuse slang or the passive voice, you may find some of the "hits" useful but be sure to make your own choice of replacement phrases. A few of the explanations may be useful. But nothing can substitute for your own judgement.

- check that all your **sources are cited correctly** in the text.

- check the **numbering sequence of your tables and figures.**

- check the **Literature Cited** for completeness and correct format.

- check the **line spacing between headings and text**, and Tables and Figures and text.

- check the **page breaks** to make sure you do not split tables or figures.

- are the **authors' names** spelled correctly?

- run spell check on the document to find **typographical errors** and read carefully for **spelling** and **grammatical errors**.

- check your main headings and subheadings for proper case and placement.

Get feedback on your manuscript and then revise your manuscript again

Getting feedback is one of the most important things that you can do to improve your article. First, be sure your co-authors have had a chance to read and comment on the draft. Then, when it is ready, give the manuscript to some colleagues. Indicate to when you would like to receive their comments, and what levels of information you would like (e.g., comments on the science, logic, language, and/or style). After you get their comments, revise your manuscript to address their concerns. Do not submit your manuscript until you feel it is ready for publication. Once it is accepted, further changes in your manuscript will be difficult and may also be costly.

Final Revision & Final Check

If possible, have your reviewer examine the paper again one last time. For PI courses, this is the opportunity for co-authors to check the final draft to make sure it satisfies their expectations. If all the changes have been made to everyone's satisfaction, make one last check of overall appearance of the document to catch recalcitrant page breaks, etc.

Check table and figure number and their text citation. Sometimes it happens that table and figure are there, but they are not cited in-text, you forget it. Do not do this thing. Finalize abstract and check the accuracy of the abstract. Lastly finalize the title and see the accuracy alphabet by alphabet.

Further Readings

- https://libguides.usask.ca/writing-help/disciplines/humanities-social-sciences

- Writing for Scholarly Journals, Publishing in the Arts, Humanities and Social Sciences, https://www.gla.ac.uk/media/media_41223_en.pdf

- Borja A, Writing the first draft of your science paper — some dos and don'ts, https://www.elsevier.com/connect/writing-a-science-paper-some-dos-and-donts

- https://www.springer.com/gp/authors-editors/journal-author/journal-author-academy
- https://www.apa.org/pubs/authors/new-author-guide.pdf
- https://projects.ncsu.edu/labwrite/index.html
- Maxim S. Pshenichnikov, Academic skills, file:///C:/Users/DELL/Desktop/Writing-paper-SEPOMO3.pdf

References

- Faber J, Writing scientific manuscripts: most common mistakes, Dental Press J Orthod. 2017; 22(5): 113–117. doi: 10.1590/2177-6709.22.5.113-117.sar
- Ohwovoriole AE, Writing biomedical manuscripts part I: fundamentals and general rules.West Afr J Med. 2011 May-Jun; 30(3):151-7.
- Ohwovoriole AE, West Afr J Med. Writing biomedical manuscripts part II: standard elements and common errors. 2011 Nov-Dec; 30(6):389-99.
- https://writingcenter.unc.edu/tips-and-tools/scientific-reports/

CHAPTER 6

Submission & Avoiding Rejections

As discussed earlier, research paper writing has the following crucial and equally important components.

1. Planning
2. Writing
3. Editing & Revising
4. Submitting Manuscript & Follow-ups
5. Avoiding Rejection

We had discussed the steps from planning to revising. Now let us move to submission and post-submission steps for review and research paper writing.

Submitting Manuscript & Follow-ups

Once you have prepared the final version of the manuscript, you should send the manuscript to the editor of the journal as earlier as possible. The following steps are needed for the same.

Identifying the mode of submission

First, identify whether you want to send the manuscript online or offline. The online submission has got its vital advantages over normal postal submission. Online submission is economical, reliable and provides for quick response in processing. If a journal has both the option opened, then one must go for the online submission. In case of offline or postal submission, provide good quality prints of the manuscript in the required number of copies. **Staple** your pages; don't use a bulky binding or cover.

Preparing a Cover Letter

Include a cover page giving the title of your paper, the name of the course, your name, the date, and the instructor's name. Don't bother with coloured paper, fancy print, or decorations. Prepare a simple, short but effective cover letter for the manuscript submission addressing the editor of the journal. Try to address the editor by his name (Dear Prof. Murthy) rather than writing just "DEAR EDITOR". It has its own impact.

Providing required information or forms

Most of the journals require the submission of a copyright form/undertaking by the author(s) in the standard format prescribed by the journal itself. In the case of papers with the inclusion of *in vivo* studies, permission taken from the animal ethical committee is also submitted, or an undertaking is submitted that concerned permission was taken by the authors from the concerned committee.

Submitting the manuscript to the editor

Follow the Instructions to Authors to determine what items you need to submit, how to submit them, and to whom you should send them. Note that some journals permit (or even require) a "peer-reviewer" be advised or proposed by the author. At this point, you may wish to list possible reviewers (or individuals to be avoided). If necessary, contact the editor to be sure that the manuscript was received. And if, after a month, you have not received a response concerning the acceptability of your manuscript for publication, you may wish to contact the editor about this, too.

Prepare the final checklist.

Check out every file. Be ready with the following files and follow these steps.

- Copyright agreement.
- Cover page.

- Title page
- Manuscript file
- Author details suggested reviewers.
- Image files or graphics.
- Before submitting your file.
- Choose your submission type/system. Sometimes it is also defined (just copy from your manuscript)
- Preview it.
- Click upload for uploading it (if satisfied with preview)
- And submit it finally.

Dealing with reviewers' comments

Most manuscripts are not accepted on the first submission. However, you may well be invited to resubmit a revised manuscript. If you chose to do so, you would need to respond to the reviewer comments. Do this with tact. Answer every concern of the reviewers and indicate where the corresponding changes were made in the manuscript if they were, indeed, made. You do not need to make all the changes that the reviewer recommended, but you do need to provide a convincing rationale for any changes that you did not make.

Once you are clear on the changes to be made, approach the revision using the same *global, paragraph, line editing* strategy.

- Make the global changes first and recheck the items listed previously.
- Make the paragraph level changes and recheck the list.
- Make the line edit changes and recheck the list.
- Recheck the miscellaneous items

When you resubmit the manuscript, indicate in your cover letter that this is a revised version.

An alternative is to submit the manuscript to another journal. However, if you do so, it may still be best to take the reviewer comments into consideration. Even if you feel that the reviewers have misunderstood something in your paper, others might do the same. Of course, if you submit to another journal, you probably will need to modify the format. And please note: You may *not* submit your manuscript to more than one journal at a time!

Plan the response/ rebuttal letter

Plan the rebuttal letter/ response to the comment letter, addressing the editor. Mentioning your article number, you will write that you are giving the response to comments. However, you will be inserting those comments/ modifying your manuscript in the word file in track changes so that each change is visible to the reviewer or editor. A file must be maintained. In a word file, you will mention the response to comments humbly, assertively and professionally.

Checking the proofs

Once the manuscript is accepted and prepared for print, the publisher will send the corresponding author page proofs of the article. This may be accompanied by a list of queries, such as missing information regarding a reference. The proofs may be sent via email or as a hard copy. If there is a chance that you will be away when the proofs arrive, have a plan for making certain that they are received, and you are notified. You may only have 24-48 hr to return the proofs.

Carefully correct any typos and factual errors. And read the manuscript for clarity – this is your last chance! However, try to limit changes to editorial queries plus minor modifications. If you think anything more major is required, you must first get permission from the journal editor and be prepared for additional costs and publication delays.

Publication

After publication, you can add the paper to your dissertation and/or thesis. This improves the acceptability and credibility of your research work. And of course, it increases the weight of your biodata also.

Please do remember, the use of publication in your thesis, which is out of your thesis work, is not considered self- plagiarism. Self-plagiarism (also termed as text-recycling without citation of your own original resource) has been discussed in the previous section of the book in an exclusive chapter of plagiarism.

Avoiding Rejection

You prepare an article with great patience, focusing and practice but even then, if it is rejected, it breaks the nerves. So, we are providing the means by which chances of rejection of articles can be minimized or avoided.

Understand Editorial Process

Only when a manuscript is matching with the scope of a journal and is complying with the formatting guidelines of the journal, it is processed for peer review. Most journals assign an editor who is responsible for processing of each submission. The editor is supported by a group of associate editors and/or reviewers.

When an article is received, most editors check the manuscript for it's adherence to Journal's guidelines. If it is complying the guidelines then only the manuscript is processed for further review to associate editors or reviewers. At this stage, the editor assesses the suitability of the manuscript for the specific journal. They also look for a minimum level of readability and checks the appropriateness of methods utilized. If the manuscript is unacceptable, the editor returns it to the author. In most cases, however, the article is forwarded to one or more associate editors for their detailed review.

Upon receipt, the associate editor reviews the manuscript in conformance with predetermined standards or publication criteria. Generally, the associate editor evaluates the manuscript in the following areas:

- Importance, timeliness, relevance of the topic to therapeutic recreation;
- Adequacy of the rationale and/or literature review;
- Logical organization of ideas and thoroughness of presentation;
- Correlation between the questions or issues investigated and implications/conclusions stated
- Clarity and consistency of writing.

In most cases, the associate editor selects several reviewers who in turn are sent the article for evaluation. The associate editor, however, usually has the same right as the editor to send poorly developed manuscripts back without further review. When reviews are received, the associate editors will combine the various reviews into a recommendation to the editor regarding disposition of the manuscript. Most journals use some variation of the following set of categories:

- Consider for publication (with minimum revisions);
- Consider for publication (with major revisions);
- Ask for major revisions before further publication consideration; or,
- Reject article.

Having received the manuscript and recommendations back from the associate editor, the editor combines the comments and recommendations from the various reviews and also places the manuscript in one of the above categories. Sometimes the author is asked to make substantial revisions before a publication decision is made. Few manuscripts are published as originally submitted. Most require some degree of revision and if these revisions are substantial, a second round of reviews will be necessary.

Avoiding Difficulties

The review process is fairly straightforward. But still author can improve the chances of acceptance by taking some steps.

Authors should focus on the following points during manuscript preparation to avoid the rejection.

- Irrelevant topic
- Lack of novelty
- Unclear/misleading argumentation
- Lack of focus (misconnection between objectives to methodology objectives to conclusions),
- Weak methodology

Conceptualization

An effective start is the utmost important aspect of a good manuscript. Many articles sound similar in presentation. For example, "The purpose of this article is to study this aspect, so I collected some data and here is what I found."

Never skip clarifying the basic concept of the study. The background information or the literature review on the topic must be provided in condensed and complete manner.

Any article must effectively provide the background and then develop the idea. Many authors fail to grab the attention in the concept development stage. An author must ascertain the theoretical basis of the study or discussion. For example, when we are talking about hair growth promotion study it may be started with the importance of the research as a psychosocial importance of the topic.

The status of research work in literature must be thoroughly discussed without any bias and then the research gap must be identified. Then a concrete problem definition followed by author's hypothesis must be presented. The aim and objectives must cater to fill the research gap. We cannot keep the readers in dark about the rational of the study.

Effective presentation Style

Sometimes even a very good study can be rejected for publication simply due to poor presentation and/or organization of the material. The poor writing style and lack cohesion and coherence in the content may be the reasons of rejections.

The editors or reviewers do not have time to improve your writing or modify the content written carelessly. Editor or reviewers often reject even the novel studies if they are not drafted effectively. Reviewers just do not want to struggle in understanding the authors writing.

Many journals also provide the assistance to authors in preparing a quality manuscript. Most of the publishers have their own author support systems. Many features of the author support systems are free. But some of the premium services are available only on payment basis. In general, journals publish a guide to article preparation or recommend a particular guide to follow.

Lastly, here are some suggestions for improving a manuscript:

- Present the article in simple language with clarity.
- Rational of the study must be clear and be focused in the entire study.
- Aims and methodology should be clearly explained.
- Provide the results systematically and in totality.
- Discuss the results critically and with logical reasoning without any general and vague statements.
- Conclude the study as per the objective of the study and provide the scope of further study required (of any) and
- Provide the supplementary data or spectra also in support of our study.
- Always stick to manuscript guidelines prescribed by the journal with respect to formatting and all other aspects of the research article.

Further Readings

- https://libguides.usask.ca/writing-help/disciplines/humanities-social-sciences

- Writing for Scholarly Journals, Publishing in the Arts, Humanities and Social Sciences, https://www.gla.ac.uk/media/media_41223_en.pdf

- Borja A, Writing the first draft of your science paper — some dos and don'ts, https://www.elsevier.com/connect/writing-a-science-paper-some-dos-and-donts

- https://www.springer.com/gp/authors-editors/journal-author/journal-author-academy

- https://www.apa.org/pubs/authors/new-author-guide.pdf

- https://projects.ncsu.edu/labwrite/index.html

- Maxim S. Pshenichnikov, Academic skills, file:///C:/Users/DELL/Desktop/Writing-paper-SEPOMO3.pdf

References

- Faber J, Writing scientific manuscripts: most common mistakes, Dental Press J Orthod. 2017; 22(5): 113–117. doi: 10.1590/2177-6709.22.5.113-117.sar

- Ohwovoriole AE, Writing biomedical manuscripts part I: fundamentals and general rules.West Afr J Med. 2011 May-Jun; 30(3):151-7.

- Ohwovoriole AE, West Afr J Med. Writing biomedical manuscripts part II: standard elements and common errors. 2011 Nov-Dec; 30(6):389-99.

- https://writingcenter.unc.edu/tips-and-tools/scientific-reports/

CHAPTER 7

Plagiarism & Ethics in Publications

Ethical practice is essential in every kind of academic activity. Any violation of basic ethics will affect the value and credibility of the activity being carried out, whether it is teaching or research or administration. The earlier professional achievement was rendered as a function of position and content only. But now, the professional achievement is rendered as a function of position, content, and ethics.

Different areas of academics may have their own detailed and specific codes of ethics, but the essence of those guidelines should be aligned.

Academic integrity

As per UGC (Promotion of academic integrity and prevention of plagiarism in higher educational institutions) Regulations, 2018 "Academic Integrity" is the intellectual honesty in proposing, performing and reporting any activity, which leads to the creation of intellectual property.

- Basic Ethics
- Scientific Conduct: (scientific misconduct, falsification, fabrication and plagiarism, redundant publications, selective reporting)
- Publication Ethics
- Teaching-learning integrity, determination & dedication
- Evaluation integrity
- Misc.

Plagiarism

As per UGC regulation 2018, "Plagiarism" means the practice of taking someone else's work or idea and passing them as one's own.

Plagiarism is academic/literary theft (intentionally or unintentionally). Plagiarism occurs when someone uses other person's language, ideas, or any other type of text material, figure and graph, which do not belong to common original knowledge without its acknowledgement.

You should not take or reproduce any theory, idea or any other study material of another person without acknowledgement. You must acknowledge the source, in each case, whether directly quoting, borrowing facts, paraphrasing of using other person's idea.

We must understand that academic writing demands zero tolerance towards plagiarism and that it is a criminal offence to steal the work of another person. Also, it should be well understood that there are serious consequences of plagiarism. If you are a faculty member, you may be suspended from the job/ concerned designation, and you will not be allowed to be a supervisor for a PhD student. And if you are a student, your registration as PhD student may be cancelled, and overall it depends on how seriously you have committed this offence. Please search and explore the various case studies of plagiarism.

UGC Regulation 2018

UGC (Promotion of academic integrity and prevention of plagiarism in higher educational institutions) Regulations, 2018 provides the regulatory framework for prevention of plagiarism with the objective to preserve academic integrity and prevent plagiarism in higher educational institutes (Fig. 1 & 2).

रजिस्ट्री सं० डी० एल०-33004/99 REGD. NO. D. L.-33004/99

भारत का राजपत्र

The Gazette of India

असाधारण

EXTRAORDINARY

भाग III—खण्ड 4

PART III—Section 4

प्राधिकार से प्रकाशित

PUBLISHED BY AUTHORITY

सं. 287] नई दिल्ली, मंगलवार, जुलाई 31, 2018/श्रावण 9, 1940

No. 287] NEW DELHI, TUESDAY, JULY 31, 2018/ SHRAVANA 9, 1940

विश्वविद्यालय अनुदान आयोग

अधिसूचना

विश्वविद्यालय अनुदान आयोग (उच्चतर शिक्षा संस्थानों में अकादमिक सत्यनिष्ठा एवं साहित्यिक चोरी की रोकथाम को प्रोत्साहन) विनियम, 2018

नई दिल्ली, 23 जुलाई, 2018

मि. सं. 1–18/2010 (सीपीपी-II).—

प्रस्तावना

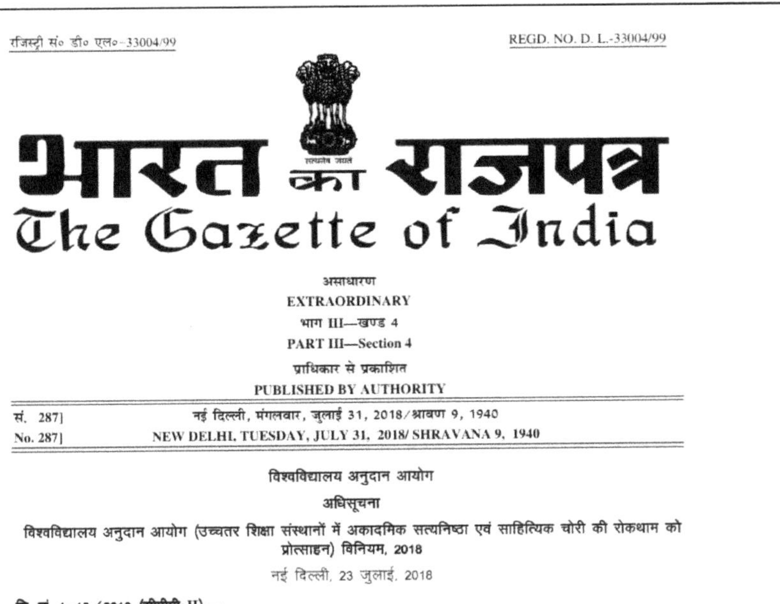

Fig. 1. The UGC regulation 2018 (https://www.ugc.ac.in/pdfnews/7771545_academic-integrity-Regulation2018.pdf)

[भाग III–खण्ड 4] भारत का राजपत्र : असाधारण 9

3. Objectives

3.1 To create awareness about responsible conduct of research, thesis, dissertation, promotion of academic integrity and prevention of misconduct including plagiarism in academic writing among student, faculty, researcher and staff.

3.2 To establish institutional mechanism through education and training to facilitate responsible conduct of research, thesis, dissertation, promotion of academic integrity and deterrence from plagiarism.

3.3. To develop systems to detect plagiarism and to set up mechanisms to prevent plagiarism and punish a student, faculty, researcher or staff of HEI committing the act of plagiarism.

4. Duties of HEI:

Every HEI should establish the mechanism as prescribed in these regulations, to enhance awareness about responsible conduct of research and academic activities, to promote academic integrity and to prevent plagiarism.

5. Awareness Programs and Trainings:

(a) HEI shall instruct students, faculty, researcher and staff about proper attribution, seeking permission of the author wherever necessary, acknowledgement of source compatible with the needs and specificities of disciplines and in accordance with rules, international conventions and regulations governing the source.

(b) HEI shall conduct sensitization seminars/ awareness programs every semester on responsible conduct of research, thesis, dissertation, promotion of academic integrity and ethics in education for students, faculty,

Fig. 2. Objectives of UGC regulation 2018.

The regulation emphasizes the sensitization of the institutes towards plagiarism and to make the mechanism to prevent the same. The regulation defines the exclusion criteria for similarity checks and quantified the plagiarism in 04 levels (Fig. 3)

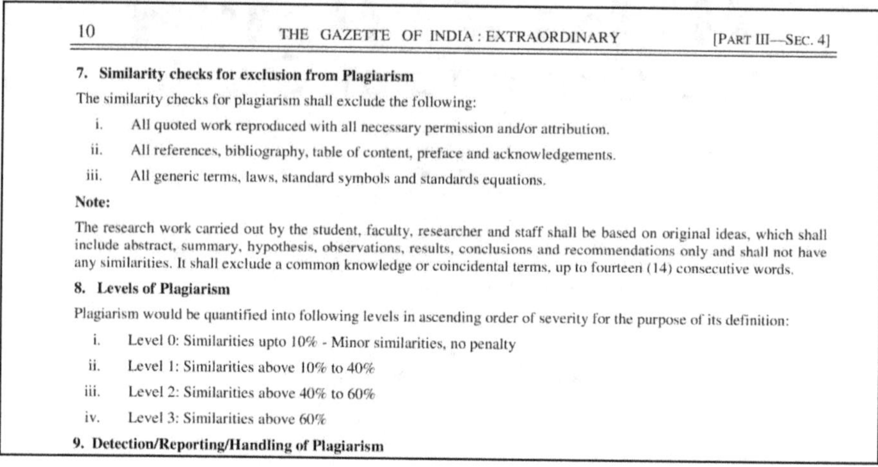

10 THE GAZETTE OF INDIA : EXTRAORDINARY [PART III—SEC. 4]

7. Similarity checks for exclusion from Plagiarism

The similarity checks for plagiarism shall exclude the following:

i. All quoted work reproduced with all necessary permission and/or attribution.

ii. All references, bibliography, table of content, preface and acknowledgements.

iii. All generic terms, laws, standard symbols and standards equations.

Note:

The research work carried out by the student, faculty, researcher and staff shall be based on original ideas, which shall include abstract, summary, hypothesis, observations, results, conclusions and recommendations only and shall not have any similarities. It shall exclude a common knowledge or coincidental terms, up to fourteen (14) consecutive words.

8. Levels of Plagiarism

Plagiarism would be quantified into following levels in ascending order of severity for the purpose of its definition:

i. Level 0: Similarities upto 10% - Minor similarities, no penalty

ii. Level 1: Similarities above 10% to 40%

iii. Level 2: Similarities above 40% to 60%

iv. Level 3: Similarities above 60%

9. Detection/Reporting/Handling of Plagiarism

Fig. 3. Exclusion criteria for similarity checks and levels of plagiarism.

The regulation recommends the establishment of the Departmental Academic Integrity Panel (DAIP) in every HEI. The regulation provides the provision of penalties to the students and faculty members who are found guilty of plagiarism. Here are three tiers of penalty for the plagiarism offence for students and faculty members as per the similarity per cent (Table 1).

Table 1 Penalties as per UGC Regulation 2018

Level	Similarity	A penalty in the submission of thesis and dissertations	A penalty in case of academic and research publications
0	up to 10%	Minor Similarities, no penalty	Minor Similarities, no penalty
1	above 10% to 40%	Such student shall be asked to submit a revised script within a stipulated time period not exceeding 6 months.	Shall be asked to withdraw the manuscript
2	above 40% to 60%	Such student shall be debarred from submitting a revised script for a period of one year.	• Shall be asked to withdraw the manuscript. • Shall be denied a right to one annual increment.

Table 1 *Contd...*

Level	Similarity	A penalty in the submission of thesis and dissertations	A penalty in case of academic and research publications
			• Shall not be allowed to be a supervisor to any new Master's, M.Phil., PhD. Student/scholar for a period of two years.
3	above 60%	Such student registration for that programme shall be cancelled.	• Shall be asked to withdraw the manuscript. • Shall be denied a right to two successive annual increments. • Shall not be allowed to be a supervisor to any new Master's, M.Phil., PhD. Student/scholar for a period of three years.

As per the regulation, "On repeated plagiarism - Shall be asked to withdraw manuscript and shall be punished for the plagiarism of one level higher than the lower level committed by him/her. In the case where plagiarism of the highest level is committed, then the punishment for the same shall be operative. In case of level 3 offence is repeated then the disciplinary action including suspension/termination as per service rules shall be taken by the HEI."

Types of plagiarism

There are four broad ways of classifying types of plagiarism.

Direct Plagiarism

Direct plagiarism is when there is a word-to-word transcription of a paragraph without the use of quotation marks or attribution. That means passing it completely or partially as his or her own work without attribution is direct plagiarism. Using another person's work is unethical, academic misconduct, and it makes grounds for disciplinary actions if caught as consequences of plagiarism may be very dangerous.

Mosaic Plagiarism (Patch writing)

Mosaic Plagiarism is borrowing phrases from any source without using quotation marks or trying to find synonyms for the author's language, keeping in view that the centric meaning of the text should not change. It is also called "patchwriting". This kind of paraphrasing, whether you do it intentionally or unintentionally, is academic misconduct. And it is punishable even if you footnote your source.

Self-Plagiarism

Self-plagiarism is when a student reuses his or her own previous work or mixes parts of previous works without permission from each and every co-author involved.

For example, Self-plagiarism is when you are incorporating a part of your paper written at your graduation level into a paper you are going to write in your post-graduation. Self-plagiarism is about taking repeated advantage of one single work…it is like using one research work for taking two degrees, or in another way, you cannot copy figures /table or some text from your previous publication for the new manuscript. Technically you have to take the permission for reproducing the content…. Otherwise, it would be treated as self-plagiarism. UGC has termed self-plagiarism "text recycling". Refer UGC public notice on clarification of self-plagiarism (Self-plagiarism: https://www.ugc.ac.in/pdfnews/2284767_self-plagiarism001.pdf)

Accidental Plagiarism

Accidental plagiarism occurs when you are busy doing literature work…and you just neglect to cite the sources or misquotes their sources, or unintentionally paraphrases a source by using similar words, groups of words without attribution. Students should learn how to cite and should practice careful noting of the sources you have used (should develop note-taking hobbit). It means be careful in noting down the tiny things you do. For example, you have taken few lines from a book, and the book is misplaced……then there may be a problem in referencing, and you could have avoided this if you have already noted the reference of the book.

Detecting Plagiarism

Plagiarism detection is done by the comparison of the Similarity of submitted literature by the author with the available literature on the local or global level.

Different tools of plagiarism detection

- iThenticate
- Plagiarism Checker X

- Turnitin
- Viper
- Grammarly
- CitePlag
- Plagiarisma.net
- ProWritingAid
- MOSS (Measure of Software Similarity)
- DupliChecker
- PaperRater
- Copyleaks
- Search Engine Reports
- PlagTracker
- Plagium
- Prepostseo

Avoiding plagiarism

Plagiarism can be avoided simply by giving due credit to the source from wherever you have taken it. So, we can say that the single key is "JUST BE HONEST".

- Give credit, attribute, cite, acknowledge the source honestly.
- Ask for permission for the use of documents and graphs.
- Respect IPR and other people's ideas
- Focus on the time points
- Anticipate the time points of academic writing where the plagiarism may remain unattended
- Refer to good quality, reliable resources in a literature survey
- Keep a record of each and every source.
- Arrange/ Organize the literature for future use

Some more points

- Put quotation marks
- Complete reframing of text is required when paraphrasing. Don't just simply rearrange sentences or replace a few words in a sentence.

- Check your rewritten version against the original version
- Form your own ideas and opinions about different issues,
- Compare voices/ides of authors and deduce your own idea/voice
- Correcting plagiarism
- Run the plagiarism checker
- See the similarity report
- Focus on the portion, which shows a high percentage of copying first.
- The per cent copying from a single source must be reduced on priority
- The results and discussion portion must be free from any plagiarism on priority.
- Introduction is generally giving the background, so chances of plagiarism are high, so focus on the correction

Plagiarism avoiding/Correcting strategies

A. Avoiding text plagiarism

- Direct Quotation
- Paraphrasing
- Summarizing

B. Avoiding image plagiarism

- Draw yourself the same with different colors
- Modify and include your idea
- Never copy result figures.
- Use software to redraw the figures

Avoiding text plagiarism

Text plagiarism can be avoided by effective use of language for better understanding and clarity of content. We must give due credit to the source. We must respect the intellectual property right of scholars honestly. Care must be taken to cite all the references listed as and when required precisely as per the style recommended.

Direct Quotation

Direct Quotation is a quote is a word, sentence, or sentences that a writer copies exactly from a source. One can quote directly by providing a reference. The direct quote also involves verbatim copying (for copying official definition and unavoidable quotes). But it's always better to paraphrase /summarize rather than directly quoting.

Let us see what the conditions are where one has to use quotes only -

- Official/ Pharmacopeial definitions/ legal language
- Unique and cannot be paraphrased without changing the meaning.
- Already clear and condensed.
- Creating a particular effect (poetry, inspiring quote) and addressing special context and author's opinion/ prestige/ aura

"But never overuse the direct quotes."

Paraphrasing

A restatement in your own words of someone else's ideas is called paraphrasing. Paraphrasing is not just changing a few words of the original sentences. It requires a complete reframing of sentences that have your own voice and your own understanding (about the author's idea). Correct and accurate paraphrasing requires highly-developed writing skills. So you have change both the words and the sentence structure of the original without changing the contextual meaning. Never forget to attribute the source, and citation is required.

Summarizing

"Reducing the source text to its main points." This avoids the overuse of direct quotations and large paraphrasing sections of the original text. Focus is on own understanding and presenting in your own words. But you still need to acknowledge the source of information, add your own comments to show your analysis and interpretation of the work.

Referencing

Learn proper referencing method/ style even down to the positioning of commas and full-stops. Referencing is to be done with every previous method of avoiding text plagiarism.

Remember various common writing or citation styles like BIG THREE "CMS, MLA, APA". Adopt the style as per your subject area and recommendation of your department/institute/ journal.

Avoiding image plagiarism

- Draw yourself the same with different colors
- Use and search free to reuse figures.

- Search Wikipedia/Wikimedia and other free to reuse resources
- Use the advanced google search/ filter for free to reuse figures.
- Modify and include your idea
- Use figure drawing software or tools like www.lucidchart.com, google drawing, MS Office tool: SmartArt etc.

Ask for permission to reproduce even it is your own figure in any other journal until you own the copyright. Never copy result figures. It may lead to retraction of paper and serious consequences.

Let's summarize some key points.

- Just be honest
- Always acknowledge, attribute and cite reference honestly.
- Use a direct quote, paraphrasing and summarizing along with proper citation of reference for avoiding text plagiarism.
- Learn the proper referencing style.
- Avoid image plagiarism by using advanced filters and redraw images manually or by software/ tools.

Further Reading

- Plagiarism - Why students do it and how you can help, https://www.youtube.com/watch?v=oCT7iamerdo
- Academic Integrity – Plagiarism,https://www.youtube.com/watch?v=MDFHd_31e_o
- How to avoid plagiarism and turnitin, https://www.youtube.com/watch?v=RrPU_bFBeF8
- https://antiplagiarism.net/blogs/avoid-plagiarism-tool/
- UNIVERSITY GRANTS COMMISSION (PROMOTION OF ACADEMIC INTEGRITY AND PREVENTION OF PLAGIARISM IN HIGHER EDUCATIONAL INSTITUTIONS) REGULATIONS, 2018 New Delhi, the 23rd July, 2018, https://www.ugc.ac.in/pdfnews/7771545_academic-integrity-Regulation2018.pdf
- Self plagiarism defined by UGC: Self-plagiarism: https://www.ugc.ac.in/pdfnews/2284767_self-plagiarism001.pdf
- Guidance Document "Good Academic Research Practices"; Sept. 2020, https://www.ugc.ac.in/ebook/UGC_GARP_2020_Good%20Academic%20Research%20Practices.pdf

References

- Gipp, Bela (2014), Citation-based plagiarism detection, Springer Vieweg Research, ISBN 978-3-658-06393-1
- Correct and accurate paraphrasing, http://www.academicintegrity.uoguelph.ca/
- http://isites.harvard.edu/icb/icb.do?keyword=k70847&tabgroupid=icb.tabgroup108986
- Kumar PM, Priya NS, Musalaiah S, Nagasree M, Knowing and avoiding plagiarism during scientific writing. Ann Med Health Sci Res. 2014 Sep;4(Suppl 3):S193-8. doi: 10.4103/2141-9248.141957.
- https://www.wikihow.com/Use-Simple-Words-in-Technical-Writing
- Debnath J. Plagiarism: A silent epidemic in scientific writing - Reasons, recognition and remedies. Med J Armed Forces India. 2016 Apr; 72(2):164-7. Epub 2016 Apr 16.
- https://www.um.edu.mt/__data/assets/pdf_file/0018/261324/avdplagiarism.pdf
- https://elearningindustry.com/top-10-free-plagiarism-detection-tools-forteachers
- https://lutow.acim56.info/a1252/

SECTION II

Thesis/ Dissertation Execution & Writing

CHAPTER 8

Introducing Research

Introduction

Research has always been the driving force of humanity. The humanity is progressing just due to constant research endeavors being undertaken by human being. Think, had the ape man not invented fire or the wheel, we would never have been here today in this status. So, the research and development are a constantly demanded process in each time. Doing research is just not passing some papers, doing some work, write the same and submit, it is more of a commitment. It is a commitment towards the sustained development of society, nation, world, and the world of science.

Doing research is a passion. This is not the field for the people who believe in getting the results overnight. The research needs patience, hard work, determination, and dedication. It is not a task with predetermined results. Many a times the outcomes may be depressive than being impressive. But never lose the patience. Thomas A. Edison said *""I will not say I failed 1000 times; I will say that I discovered there are 1000 ways that can cause failure."*

The importance of research has faced a quantum change in the post GATT era. After signing the WTO's GATT agreement, India has entered in the product patent era. Now the new products and new inventions are the vital need of any industry. Pharma Industries which were not investing more than 2-5 % of their turnover in R&D before 1995, started to invest in double digits in R&D. The run/competition for doing invention, getting patents and marketing innovative products has boost up the R&D. But still today industries and academia are working in isolation with respect to R&D. Unlike in western countries where industrial and academic interaction is strong, India does not have such close partnership for R&D between industry and academia. However, the policy makers are talking much about this now. But the results are yet to come.

The National Education Policy (NEP) 2020 has also emphasized on developing a vibrant research environment in higher educational Institutions. NEP has made the provision to develop research Universities, National Research Foundation and to promote multidisciplinary research.

In the present section we shall be focusing on the academic research [specially done to get the Ph D and master's degree in science subjects (Life sciences, Chemistry, Physics, Pharmacy etc.) and management] and thesis writing. You can easily link the discussion of various points with your own area.

(a) Types of research studies

In the multi disciplinary era of research, no research is confined as such to a single type. But still grossly research may be of following three types.

- Exploratory Studies

   Defined as *"Preliminary research conducted to increase understanding of a concept, to clarify the exact nature of the problem to be solved, or to identify important variables to be studied."*

- Descriptive Studies

   Defined as *"Descriptive research studies answer the, who what, where, when and how questions. It is used when one wants to gain a better understanding of the specifics or details the research issue."*

- Causal Studies

   Defined as *"Research studies that examine whether the value of one variable cause or determines the value of another variable."*

Each of the above type of research has different purpose and key methods (Table 1).

Table 1 Various Types of research studies, purpose, and methods

Type of Study	Purpose	Key Methods
Exploratory Studies	• Define Terms • Clarify Problems • Develop Theories • Establish Priorities • Gain General Information	• Pilot Studies • Focus Groups • Case Analyses • Secondary Data • Concept Testing • Depth Interviews • Taste Tests • Experience Surveys
Descriptive Studies	• Confirm Theories • Brand Loyalty Measure • Describes Population • Build Customer Profile • Gain Specific Information	• Secondary Data • Cross sectional Surveys • Longitudinal Surveys • Statistical Data Analysis
Causal Studies	• Confirm Theories • Identify Cause & Effect Relationships Among Variables	• Surveys • Experiments • Time Sequence • Secondary Data • Systematic Elimination

(b) Selection of a Research Method

A research employs any of the following methods for getting to its goals or hypothesis.

- **Observation Research:**

  Typically, descriptive research that monitors respondents' actions without direct interaction

- **Experiments:**

  Research to measure causality, in which the researcher changes one or more variables and observes the effect of the changes on another variable.

- **Survey Research:**

  It is the research in which an interviewer interacts with respondents to obtain facts, opinions, and attitudes.

- **Other Qualitative Research:**

  It is the research dealing with focus groups, interviews, secondary analysis, and case studies.

However, research methodology itself is a broad subject to study. This includes various theories, models and techniques used as the tool to conduct or analyze the research and its results e.g., Critical Path Method, simplex, etc.

Drug discovery research are very complex. The following table provides the various approaches of drug discovery research.

Table 2 Various approaches of drug discovery research

Approach	Key Methods
Traditional	• Trial and error • Diverse cultures and systems of medicines e.g., morphine, quinine, ephedrine, and artemisinin (anti-malarial)
Empirical	• Builds on understanding of relevant physiological process • Use of naturally occurring lead molecule e.g., tubocurarine, quinine and cocaine
Molecular I	• Most drug discovery is based on this approach • Molecular biological techniques • Advances in genomics
Molecular II	• Random screening Pragmatic and dominant at present • Rational drug design Computer-assisted techniques • Anti-sense approach Manipulation of genetic targets

Molecular III	• Technological Developments:
	• High throughputs of potential compounds
	   o Molecular biological knowledge
	   o Instrumentation
	   o Information Technology
	   o Screening

(c) Challenges in academic research and student projects

Except a few states of art academic institutes, academic research is not taken very seriously in India. There are various challenges in developing a solid background for research environment.

The availability of resources for research work (like infrastructure, analytical equipments, technical manpower and faculty members experienced in performing research projects) is the prime challenge in development of research environment in an academic institute.

As far as the M. Pharm. research projects are concerned the quality of M. Pharm research projects is going down with the mushroom growth of institutes which only aim for making profits. Students are in hurry to finish up their projects and getting jobs just after their submission. The students do not even want to spend the minimum time of one year assigned to perform the research projects. In past the M. Pharm course was of one and half year duration. But it was extended up to two years with the aim of emphasizing the research part. This extension provided a full one year for research project in comparison of six-month duration in the last syllabi. But the extension could not meet the objective by and large. The institutes which were performing well turned better in view of projects' outcome. But the average institutes which aim only for profit making do not take these aspects seriously and just cater the demand of increasing the number of faculty and reducing the expenditure on projects, directly and indirectly support the students in finishing and submitting the research projects as earliest. For common mass of students, in practical terms doing and submitting the research projects has become a formality only.

A good alternative of institutional research (PG research projects or sometimes for Ph D work also) is the industrial research also. Students perform their projects in Pharmaceutical Industries. But again, the concept is not catering the actual need that is the creation of academic research environment. The industries do not permit the students to perform the research work chosen or planned by students themselves. Instead, the industries use the students as a free/honorary manpower and get the routine works (of negligible importance) of industry conducted by them. However, even if the students do some new work assigned by the industry, they are not told about the drug or polymers or any other information which they must know. So even if they do some new work, they are unaware of actual importance of the work. Moreover, the students are not allowed to publish their research findings performed in industrial setting due to binding of not revealing trade secrets. No doubt, students learn a lot about the practical industrial approach but the practice of sending students to industry for PG projects just for the sake of saving the money of chemicals and efforts from academic supervisors deprives the academic research to blossom. Students should know what best they can do out of the available resources. Most of the times, even very good research can be planned in bare limited resources. By hiring analytical services, the availability of analytical equipments can be coped with. Even the animal house facilities can be availed or shared with other institutes. The key message is outsourcing a part of research is OK but the complete shifting or moving out of the academic laboratories is not good for the health academic research.

On the other hand, Ph D degree has always been very demanding for career growth of faculty members as well as for easy entry of students in academic profession. The previous rules and regulations of appointment did not pose any obstacles for non-Ph D persons to get the higher posts in academics (Associate Professor or even Professor). But the new regulations by University Grants Commission of India (UGC) and All India Council of Technical Education (AICTE) do not allow any person to get the higher posts (except the person with industrial experience) without Ph D. The picture of increasing demand of Ph D has resulted in a race for doing the Ph D. In many states number of PG pharmacy students passing out is far more than the passing out pharmacy graduates. This is resulting in the easy availability of faculties at lecturer level but at reader and professor level it is tough to get the faculty with Ph D and teaching experience (8 years by UGC and 5 years by AICTE). A major percentage of students passing out of the PG courses prefer to do the Ph D with their academic jobs. But it is again a hurricane task to do the Ph D with the job specially for the faculty members of non-governmental academic institutes. The managements of private colleges are almost always reluctant to provide necessary leaves and other facilities to their faculty members for doing Ph D work. On the other hand, University departments or government colleges are better place to do Ph D work by faculty members with their jobs and as research fellows in projects funded by agencies like UGC, AICTE or DST. The regular faculty members of University departments may also get the research grants from UGC and AICTE to conduct the research work along with their jobs. These grants are also given to accredited private colleges by AICTE. But a very few persons get these projects. The competition is very high in this front also. Moreover, the projects are generally sanctioned after about one to two years of peer reviewing, scrutiny and other official formalities (Refer Appendix 1 for various funding agencies).

Another challenge is availability of good books and journals. The students find it hard to review the literature due to scarcity of good journals. Many a times even the internet facility is not provided to PG and Ph D students. Due to financial limitations students also are not able to refer the libraries of other state of art institutes. Moreover, students are not aware of using the internet properly for referring the journals. The students are unaware about the good impact journals which provide free full text. The free services provided by the UGC to Universities regarding availability of e journals are also under utilized in most of the Universities.

Solutions to the challenges:

- Promote doing the project in institutes
- Inculcate habit and art of referring journals
- Inculcating Team efforts among students
- Going for MOUs or other venture between institutes or departments for sharing facilities
- Aware students about hiring analytical services
- Promote students for attending conferences to generate research themes

(d) Need of doing potential need based and rational research work (developing a research environment):

In the present time, besides the research on conventional topics or basic science, the need based research are always on high priority and get accepted as the projects for governmental funding. The aim and objectives must be rational and with strong reasoning. We cannot do research for doing research only. There must be an evidence of hypothesis for expected positive outcome. As we have discussed earlier this may be exploratory or of other types. Doing basic and fundamental research (exploring a lead molecule etc.) are not well suited for short time M. Pharm. Projects. Many more potential research can be done in a short time (one year). The major works can be subdivided into various projects which in turn can be performed by different students. But each subdivided work which is made or planned as an individual work must be a complete task itself and should have its own importance. We cannot expect much from a student like doing an invention or exploring a very novel work. But at least, the concept of research methodology can be incubated during their project tenure in their brains. At least they should be capable enough to plan a new work and execute the same themselves in future.

In the present time each country and funding agencies have their own thrust areas (focus areas) of research to which they support. The recent published work can also give the essence of demand and scope of the research area. The thrust areas must be targeted for research along with the fact of availability of resources.

Thrust areas as per All India Council of technical Education (AICTE)

1. Advanced Electronics, Power Electronics, Sensors and Transducers

2. Alternate Automobile Fuels

3. Alternative Sources of Energy (Solar, Photo-voltaic/Photo-thermal, Wind, Bio,

4. Tidal, Geo-Thermal Systems)

5. Anti-Cancer Technology

6. Architecture, Urban and Regional Planning, Aspects of Environmental Degradation etc.

7. Automotive Electronics Systems

8. Bio-medical Engineering

9. Biotechnology, Genetic Engineering and Tissue Culture

10. Chemical Technology: Development of New Processes, Development/Improvement of Drugs/Pharmaceuticals, Chemicals, Petrochemicals, Fertilizers and Allied, Textile Processing

11. CNG Application

12. Coastal Zone Management

13. Computational Fluid Dynamics (CFD)

14. Computer Vision and Graphics; Multi-Media, Parallel Processing, CAD/CAM

15. Control System including Computerized Control in Industry

16. Corrosion in Structures – Cryogenics

17. Development of Fuzzy logic Technology – Disaster Mitigation

18. Education Technology

19. Environment, Atmospheric Engineering and Technology – Flexible Manufacturing Systems

20. Fluidized Bed Combustion/Pulverized Coal Combustion-Fly Ash Utilization

21. Fuel Cells

22. Futuristic materials including Fibers and Composites, Plastics & Conducting Plastics, Glass Ceramics and Electro Ceramics Superconductors

23. Global Finance

24. Herbal Drug Technology

25. Immuno-modulatory Drugs (Anti-Aids Agent)-Industrial Engineering and startup ventures.

26. Information Technology

27. Integrated Operation of Large-Scale Modern Power Systems, Information

28. System, Robotics-International Trade

29. Large Biogas Systems

30. Laser Technology

31. Low-cost Construction Technology

32. Maintenance Engineering, Reliability and Terotechnology

33. Management Information System, Management of Urban and Rural

34. Development, Human Resource Management, etc.

35. Marine Biology (Sedimentology, Oceano Temperature Gradient), Ocean S&T including Natural Products

36. Material Processing

37. Natural and man-made Hazards, Mitigation (Technological, Chemical, Nuclear, Radioactive, Environmental, Climatology) & Protection

38. Need based/Appropriate Technology for Rural and Urban Development

39. New Drug Discovery, Drug Delivery Systems, Computer Aided Drug Design,

40. Alternative Medicines, Toxicity studies

41. Non-traditional Machining Processes-NVH (Noise, Vibration & Harshness)

42. Optical Fiber Technology

43. Pavement Management and Road Safety

44. Precision Engineering, Computer Aided Eng.. (CAE)

45. Quality Engineering System and Total Quality Management (TQM)

46. Remote Sensing and Satellite Image Processing

47. Radio Frequency Planning, Advanced Radio Engineering, and Satellite

48. Communication systems including Optical Communication and ISDN

49. Smart Sensors and Intelligent Processing

50. Telematics

51. Tribology

52. Vehicular Emissions (Petrol & Diesel) – Virtual Intelligence Applications

53. Virtual Reality and Advanced Simulation

54. Waste Management, Effluent Treatment and Recycling

Thrust Areas

Pharmacy (herbal medicines):

(i) Development of drugs and formulation for primary health children and women welfare.

(ii) Microcomputers identification of indigenous drugs and development of standards.

(iii) Development of herbal medicines for chronic diseases like asthma, diabetes, rheumatism, paralysis, hypertension, skin diseases.

(iv) Development of herbal medicines for viral diseases like TB, cancer, leprosy, Aids, herpes.

(v) Development of herbal medicines for circulatory diseases like leukemia, cardiotonic, hypertension.

(vi) Screening, identification, propagation, and processing of potential medicinal plants.

(vii) Identification / investigation and formulation for personal care products.

Indian Council of Medical Research

Thrust Areas of Research

- Communicable diseases including viral diseases, cholera and enteric diseases, tuberculosis, leprosy, malaria, filariasis, kala-azar, vector control etc.

- Reproductive health including fertility control.

- Maternal & Child Health.

- Nutritional and major metabolic disorders.

- Primary health care, alternative health care systems.

- Non-communicable diseases including cancer, mental health, cardiovascular, neurological, ophthalmic, and hematological disorders, oral health, gastroenterology, urology etc.

- Occupational and other environment related health problems i.e. asthma.

- Drug research including medicinal plants and indigenous/or traditional systems of medicine.

- Basic medical research in disciplines such as anatomy, allergy, anthropology, physiology, biochemistry, immunology, cell & molecular biology, genetics, pharmacology, hematology etc.

CHAPTER 9

Planning a Topic

Planning a topic for research work is the most important task. This must be done with great care and attention. A sound preparation and planning must be done before commencing the research work. The following factors (all together) should be considered for planning a topic for research.

Preplanning

Ph D is the highest formal academic degree. It provides the maximum weight in a biodata. Therefore the planning of a topic must be done well before the actual commencement of the Course. If a student wants to do Ph D, he or she should keep this in mind before entering the third semester. The preplanning begins in the second semester or at the end of first year of post graduate course. In the second semester itself a gross idea about the field of research must be planned. And the efforts should be directed to learn the know-how of the related area. The concerned theory part must be given extra attention, so that the basic concept of the work may be cleared by students. A student can do the small experiments (as the pilot runs) of the probable topics and can then form the basis of the selection of feasible and potential topic out of those. In these experiments the student can get the close supervision and directions from a teacher and understand all the basics of the work. A carefully planned topic always results in concrete research work. PG projects can also be extended into Ph D work with inclusion of new parameters. But a Ph D title needs a more sound literature survey. The literature survey part shall be dealt in detail in subsequent sections.

Area of interest of supervisor

The supervisor's area of interest is also an important deciding factor. In his area of expertise, a supervisor can guide the students in the best possible way. First, the prospective supervisor should be consulted or asked for deciding the topic. A topic assigned by the supervisor will be more sound due to his experience in the field. Moreover, the supervisor shall be available as a ready reference during the work. However, a mutually decided new work in a new area can also be planned after careful consideration of all other factors.

Availability of resources

Every planning goes all in vain if the availability of resources is not considered. The topic of research work should be planned according to the need of its requirements and the availability of resources in the institute. The resources which are to be considered include- good literature, infrastructure/laboratory facilities, chemicals, glassware, animals and necessary equipments. For field studies availability of subjects is the main constraint. For example it is typical to do the research on the clinical consequences of anti-retroviral therapy (for AIDS patients), because the subjects are not available for any responses most of the times due to various psychosocial and other factors. If at any stage there is any feasibility to avail the facilities from other institutes or departments it must be established or confirmed well in advance. A list of requirements should be prepared and then checked for availability. If any alternatives can substitute the requirement, it should also be worked out and planned. The alternatives or changes in the topic may be planned on the directions of supervisor. Sometimes wonderful research can be planned in many deficiencies and scarcity of resources. A good planning can also pave the way for the feasibility of work.

Availability of funds is another vital resource specially for self financed research projects (by students or faculty members). AICTE has first recognized the need of supporting updating faculty members with higher education in the form of Quality Improvement Program (QIP). In

QIP, AICTE provides an opportunity to teachers teaching in diploma colleges for getting M Pharm. It also provides the opportunity to teachers teaching in B. Pharm. or M. Pharm courses to do Ph D from selected institutes. AICTE provides the full salary to the concerned faculty members during his/her leave (for Ph D) from the institute in which he or she has been working. AICTE and UGC are the funding agencies which also provide the research grants to regular faculty to conduct the research work along with their jobs in their institutes.

Availability of sophisticated or expensive services, equipments or software:

In almost every area of research analytical equipments like UV, IR, MS, NMR, HPLC and other sophisticated and expensive equipments (like DSC, XRD, SEM) and / or software (statistical software, Pharmacokinetic software etc.) are needed. The availability of these in the institute cannot form the basis (alone) of selection and decision of a topic. In general, no single institute can have all these highly expensive equipments and services in a single roof. Therefore, these kinds of services may be hired from the other academic research bodies which provide these facilities to research students by taking nominal charges (Refer Appendix 3: Directory of analytical service providers). The sophisticated analytical instrument facilities (SAIF) are provided by various SAIF labs (like in CDRI Lucknow) funded by UGC and various instrument labs in IITs. The free software can be asked/requested from the owner of the company for trial. These trial versions work well for research purposes.

Novelty of work

A research work must have sufficient elements of novelty. A sound literature and patent search can guarantee the novelty. Even if an entirely new topic is not found, the novelty can be imparted in the published or previous work by doing the work with new drugs, polymers, methods, models, or the combination thereof. The Ph D research work should be novel enough so that it can be published in high impact. This is to note that in recent guidelines (July 11, 2009, The Gazette of India) by UGC, a candidate must publish one research paper in referred journal before the submission of Ph D thesis and produce evidence for the same in the form of acceptance letter or reprint.

Time factor

The Time management is the most crucial aspect. We cannot expect a student to devote more than one year in PG projects and more than 3-5 years in Ph D research. The topic should be chosen based on its requirement of probable time span. The topic should be broad enough to keep the student indulged for the prescribed period (one year for PG project and 2 to 3 years for Ph D work). If a novel and potential topic needs more than the desired time, some parameters of study can be skipped without losing its overall importance and potential.

CHAPTER 10

Literature Survey

Sources of literature survey

As we have earlier mentioned that a sound literature search can guarantee the novelty of work. To search, collect and refer the literature need to be done in a systematic plan from standard and reliable sources. Classification of Sources: The sources of literature may be classified as followed.

Primary sources: The original thesis or data collected and presented by a researcher. E.g.: patents, Ph D thesis, research papers in journals.

Secondary sources: The original data and studies of an original study quoted or collected by another author e.g. review papers.

Tertiary sources: The primary and secondary data collected and presented by different scientists/authors e.g. edited books.

In general, we can classify the literature survey in two major classes viz Off line and On Line literature Survey.

Off line Literature survey: Literature collection should be commenced from the theory part from books and then from the research and review papers of journals available in the departmental or institutional library. Related encyclopedias and pharmacopeia should be referred for understanding the basic concepts. Referring and searching should be done with good planning. A particular journal should be taken once and all its available issues should be searched. While searching if any important article is found note down its reference (Author, title, journal, year, volume, issue, page no.). When scanning of one journal is finished then collect the issues in which articles of interest have been identified and get the articles Xeroxed. Now move to the next journal in the same way.

To refer compilation of abstracts, like Manual of Aromatic Plants Abstracts (MAPA), Indian Science Abstracts (ISA) is very helpful and timesaving. After a particular abstract of importance is identified from these, the same can be then traced from that journal's database. The project reports or previous thesis may also be consulted. This may also help in getting the cross references (references cited in text or reference in an article) which may in turn be collected further.

On Line Literature Survey: Gone are those days, when doing literature survey was a hurricane task which usually took months and sometime years. Now with the help of internet the literature search can be done in just a few days. If an institutional library has the access or subscription of SCOPUS like abstracting services the search becomes very easy. One can find every related reference in full text by just giving key words in task (search) bar of website of SCOPUS like abstracting agencies. The website of national medical library of US (www.pubmed.com) provides a very useful platform for searching the articles. This provides abstract, full text (if available free), and the link to journals associated with the key word given in task bar. Even if these services or the subscription of individual journals (on line) is not available, the search can be done through Google like search engines. But this shall provide only those articles' full text which are available free of cost. While using the search engines search should be done by changing the key words and trying again and again. Key words may be author's name, year, name of drug/plant, activity, delivery system etc. and their combinations thereof. If you are using Google search engine, then search through Google Scholar only. It shall save your time and efforts. Google scholar provides scholarly articles only and filters unnecessary sites and matter. These features can also be explored in other search engines. Other alternative is to search through publisher of journals' site (like that of Elsevier, Taylor and Francis, Bentham Science, Springer, Willey etc.) for journals of interest and then start searching the individual journal issue by issue.

Even if the full text is not available we can get the exact reference which can be collected from anywhere else.

Many good journals from reputed publishers provide full text for free. These useful journals are listed in Table 1. Nowadays Open access publishers also provide the articles free of cost (Table 2).

Table 1 List of Some pharmaceutical journals which provide free full text

S. No.	Name of Journal	Website
1.	Journal of Pharmacy and Pharmaceutical Sciences	http://www.ualberta.ca/~csps/Journals/JPPS.htm
2.	Acta Pharmaceutica	http://public.carnet.hr/acphee/
3.	Biological Pharmaceutical Bulletin	http://bpb.pharm.or.jp/
4.	Chemical Pharmaceutical Bulletin	http://cpb.pharm.or.jp/
5	AAPS PharmSciTech	www.aapspharmscitech.org
6	Pharmaceutical Technology	http://www.pharmtech.com/
7	Drug Delivery Technology	http://www.drugdeliverytech-online.com/
8	Indian Journal of Pharmaceutical Sciences	http://ijpsonline.com/
9	Indian Journal of Pharmacology	www.ijp-online.com/
10	Indian journal of Physiology of Pharmacology	www.ijpp.com/
11	Indian Journal of Pharmaceutical Education and Research	www.ijperonline.com/
12	BMC Clinical Pharmacology	http://www.biomedcentral.com/bmcclinpharmacol/
13	BMC Pharmacology	http://www.biomedcentral.com/bmcpharmacol/

Referring e Journals: Many e journals are also available which provide the free full text but are not published off line. But the mushroom growth of these kinds of journals especially in India is lowering down the standards of applied research. Many journals are also published off line also and aim for making profits by taking undue charges for paper publication and forcing the authors for subscription of the journal. In many cases of online only e journals incompetent persons deal with the manuscripts. Sometime these journals also claim their own impact factor calculated by themselves. This is very strange because it must be kept in mind that we cannot calculate the impact factor of the journal ourselves.

It is calculated on yearly basis by international indexing agencies like ISI and Thompson.

Referring State of Art Libraries: Many state of art libraries of various governmental agencies and institutes are also of vital importance for referring the national and international journals and books, both offline and online. The *list of these libraries* is given in Table 1. These libraries also provide the free access to online journals to guest users. Visiting these libraries for just a few days may solve the purpose. But these visits shall be planned after doing the previous home work by searching and identifying the exact reference as much as possible.

Table 1 List of Some libraries

S. No.	Name of Library/ institutes
1.	National Medical Library (NML)
2.	Library of NISCAIR, New Delhi
3.	University of Hyderabad Library
4.	CDRI Lucknow Library
5.	Online library of WHO (NEERI)
6.	NIPER's Library
7.	Indian Institute of Technology (IIT) Library
8.	IISC Bangalore Library
9.	IICT Hyderabad Library
10.	University of Delhi Library

Contacting authors: Many times, contacting authors for their paper is also useful. If a particular article is not available from any source, and if we know the contact address of authors we can request the full text from them by postal or e mail.

Convergent literature survey (From broad to specific topic)

The literature cannot be searched in random manner. We will have to classify our need in different topics and subtopics. Search should begin for broader area of research and then should be taken systematically to the focused area. For example if we want to do work on antidiabetic formulation development of some plants we shall search in the following sequence:- Diabetes as disease→ medicinal plants investigated for antidiabetic activity→ In vivo models for diabetes→ Herbal antidiabetic formulations→ Plant survey of selected plants→ survey of previous work done on antidiabetic activity on the selected plants.

Filing and Documentation of literature

The filling of literature collected should be well systematic and easy to access or refer. The Xerox copies of articles on a particular sub topic should be kept in a file. Alternatively the complete literature should be grouped in topics and subtopics and bound in a book form (or spiral binding) or in guard file with pagination done and an index provided in the beginning of the compilation. The indexing/list of content shall make it easy to refer the desired article. Even the copy of basic theory part from books should be there to make the literature complete in all aspect. The online files (pdf, word, ppt, html etc.) of various topics and subtopics should also be grouped in different folders and subfolders. If a matter has been copied in word file from a website, the exact URL or website of source and the date on which it was accessed should be mentioned at the end of file.

Planning review papers

If we want to understand the research topic or area completely we should plan the review paper of the topic immediately after the completion of literature survey. The planning and publication of a review forms the basis of Chapter of literature review of thesis in advance. Secondly, this prepares researcher for writing the complete thesis. Thirdly, a publication boosts the morale of researcher and increase the weight of his or her biodata. Writing a review paper is an art as well as science. The review papers should be planned very carefully. This section is separately discussed in the next chapter.

<h1>CHAPTER 11</h1>

<h1>Preparing Synopsis</h1>

If we have decided a particular topic and done the literature survey, efforts should be concentrated to prepare an outline of work. This is presented in the form a synopsis (brief research proposal) for approval of the topic from the authorities (like research degree committee). For this we should provide the following in very brief, specific, and concise manner. The length of each part of the synopsis may vary depending on the requirement of individual institutional guidelines.

Introduction

In introduction, provide background of the research area in brief. And directly move to origin of the idea or what make you think to work on the topic. This should be about one or two A4 double spaced typed pages.

Literature review

A brief review of literature covering current national and international status of the research area (and the topic specifically) should be given. The important studies should be given in brief with referencing. This part should be again of not more than two pages. Studies should be given chronologically from that of current to previous years (i.e. studies of year

2010 shall come first, then of year 2009 and so on). Until and unless the word limit or length of the part is prescribed in any guidelines, only a few important studies (about 10 to 15) should be discussed.

Aim of the study

This is the heart of the synopsis. A strong and rational reason of doing the work should be provided. The aim of the study should be clear and convincing. The language should be easy and to the point. The unnecessary elaboration of this part dilutes its importance.

"Ofloxacin hydrochloride is an anti-infective drug, used mainly in the treatment of lower respiratory infections, skin infection, urinary tract infections, and sexually transmitted diseases (except syphilis). Ofloxacin has broad activity against bacterial (Helicobacter pylori) infections and is used in combination with other drugs to treat tuberculosis. The bioavailability of ofloxacin is strongly dependent on the local physiology in the GI tract. Ofloxacin is preferably absorbed from the upper part of the gastrointestinal tract. Ofloxacin is readily soluble in the acidic environment of the stomach. In the intestine, (where neutral to slightly alkaline pH conditions prevail) precipitation of the active compound occurs, which adversely affects absorption in the lower sections of the intestine. Therefore there is a need for systems that reside in the stomach over a relatively long time and release the drug there in a sustained manner (Sen and Kshirsagar, 2002). This can be achieved by the design and development of sustained release gastroretentive floating drug delivery system for ofloxacin (using suitable polymers) which would float and deliver the drug in the upper part of GIT in a sustained manner. The present work deals with the formulation and characterization of floating microspheres of ofloxacin hydrochloride using ethyl cellulose, polyvinyl pyrrolidone K-90 (PVP K-90) and poly vinyl alcohol."
-Semalty et al. IJPSN 2010

Objectives

For minor research projects (PG projects), most of the times, objectives part is not needed in much detail. It can be said that the work is not actually too big to be subdivided in objectives like in the case PG projects. Many a times, only a single statement works well as aim as well as objective. But for the Ph D research work the aim of study should be subdivided in smaller objectives. These objectives should be SMART (Specific, Measurable, Attainable, Relevant and timebound). In totality the set of objects should meet the aim of the study. It should be set one line objectives given one after another.

Defining methodology

This is the part where the chief methodology of the work is discussed. While the aim and objective part deals with the WHAT (you are going to do?), the methodology part deals with the HOW (you are going to do it?). A brief statement of the methodology should be provided in a single stanza.

Time schedule of work

Time and work schedule should be planned. This is a simple time table of your work. This part should tell when you are going to finish a task in the entire duration and tells how the completion of a phase of the work is related with the commencement of the next phase. This is either given by CPM (Critical path method), PERT chart (Performance evaluation review technique) or by simple tabular presentation. Examples are shown as below.

References

A synopsis should have limited references depending upon the prescribed guidelines. In general a synopsis should have about 10-15 references. All references should be properly and uniformly cited in the text. The way of references writing should be uniform. Other details regarding references shall be covered in report writing section.

CHAPTER 12

Procurements & Execution of Work

All required goods must be procured on time and in sufficient quantity and quality to ensure the smooth functioning of the work.

Procurement of drugs or plants

If new drugs of good quality are needed, the source of the particular drug be identified and the purchase should be completed during literature survey or immediately after the approval of topic.

Procuring drugs through purchase from quality firms and vendors: The same chemical can be purchased on a very low cost from different vendors and firms. But quality should never be compromised. Especially when the quantitative results are to be deduced the quality chemicals should only be purchased. When the chemical are to be purchased from abroad, only known and quality firms should be selected (like Sigma Aldrich etc.). Moreover, more time frames should be allowed for procurement of these (imported) chemicals and equipments.

Procuring drugs as gift samples: The drugs can also be requested from pharmaceutical industries as gift samples. For this a nicely drafted letter should be sent to the concerned company with name and required quantity of drug. And when the drug is received as gift samples the receipt should immediately be acknowledged with gratitude and a statement about the promise to mention the acknowledgement in thesis and other publications (out of the work). This increases the probability of answering of your further request in future.

The drug sample received should be immediately identified by standard tests like melting point, FTIR, chemical assay etc.

Collection of plants: The collection of plants for study should be carefully planned and executed. The collection of plant should be done at suitable season and time from suitable location to get the maximum bioactive constituent. For example, fruits, flowers, and leaves are collected before opening/ripening, before opening buds and before reproduction starts, respectively. Sometime, the time of collection in a day should also be selected based on circadian rhythmic change in bioactive constituents. In Ayurveda also, the time of collecting a particular plant is sometime precisely defined in terms of part of a day chosen for collection (as dawn, dusk etc.). The age of plant and its geographical location also play vital role in getting maximum bioactive constituent or activity. Cinnamon is obtained in good quantity in the plants of age less than or equal to 40 yrs. The plant should never be collected from road side or any other polluted location (like near a factory, garbage dumping area etc.).

Plants and the parts thereof must be identified by the competent persons like taxonomists. The nearest botany department is the best place to get the herbs identified. Many a times the same herb is identified by matching the same with plants of herbarium maintained in the concern department and the voucher number of the herbarium is noted and mentioned for identification of the plant.

Procurement of polymers chemical, reagents solvents etc.

Polymers if expensive can be procured as gift samples from concerned companies. If you have funds quality drugs and polymers must be procured from reliable sources (like Sigma Aldrich, Merck, HiMedia etc.) yourself. The quality and grade of purchased chemicals, glassware and solvents must be ensured. It is better to identify a good and reliable vender who can supply any contingently needed items. Always use the solvents of same grade of same company throughout a particular study. This improves the reproducibility of the results.

Procurement/arrangement of animals

If you are going to perform in vivo studies the availability and health of animals should be ensured. Animals should be procured from authentic sources only (like IVRI Bareilly or other veterinary institutes or departments, NIN Hyderabad). The animals should be closely watched and cared for any disease or undesired signs. The standards of sanitation, light, water, and diet etc should be followed. Animal study protocol should be prepared and be presented before the institutional animal ethical committee for approval. The approval letter and number should be kept in record properly. These records are generally asked by the publisher of research papers (arising out of your work) with the submission of research paper.

If you are not aware of standard techniques and basic knowledge of handling the animals, do not start the animal handling just for hit and trial. This is unethical. Be sound in animal handling, get the proper and adequate training and then proceed for animal experiments.

Execution of Work

Once you have prepared everything for commencing the research work, begin the lab work step by step as planned. During the execution of you research plan you should take care of the following points.

Pilot study/run

Do not jump directly to full scale research work. Rather you should plan and execute a pilot study representing your full research work. A pilot study is generally a tiny representative work of the full study. This study should be taken up with small quantities of ingredients of work's components. The study may also be a group of hit and trial to get the desired method and materials suitable for full study. The pilot study should be planned in such a way that you can just elaborate the work and directly reach to focus area of research in full qualitative and quantitative manner. The results of pilot study should carefully be interpreted because they may also be like that due to the pilot nature of the study. The pilot runs save the time, energy, and money in clearly understanding and predicting the need of the research. This also protects researcher from any avoidable misunderstanding, confusion, and problem during full scale research. Therefore plan a small batch of work, run it and then evaluate its performance. Then prepare the list of any precaution which must be taken during the work. The preformulation aspects may also be said as a type of pilot studies. But more precisely they are the integral part of the work. But the objectives of preformulation studies are same as that of a pilot study. In case of pharmacological models, the model should be run with minimum possible of animals first, and when you are confident and clear, go ahead with the full scale study. Do not feel confident of yourself by just referring the study protocols in a published article. So many variants including the temperature, humidity, quality/grades of chemicals, type of apparatus, strains of animal, experience etc. may affect the study and result in relatively different results, even when the same protocol has been adopted.

Documentation of every task
(Do what you write and write what you do)

Whenever you are planning a new formulae, changing the formulae, modifying the method, changing grades of chemicals or any other change which is not the part of your synopsis or previous plan, note it down. Moreover, we recommend that you should prepare a daily log book of your work and should note down whatever you do. The principal of management (GMP): *"Do what you write and write what you do"* should be followed as such. Any future planning should also be noted down. Every task, reading etc. should be noted. You should also note any specific confusion or element of doubt and discuss the same with your supervisor or guide. The outcomes of discussion with supervisor should also be noted. Basically this log book should elicit the working blueprint of the research work. This notebook shall be of great help when the results are being compiled and discussed. Many a times, when you are facing some problems with results or calculations then you can pin point the problem by just going back and referring the notebook. Then the remedial measures can be taken up accordingly.

Convergent targeting to core study

The study should reach the target issue in a convergent manner. For example if you are aiming to develop some potential formulations, you should prepare the formulations in various possible and feasible ratios of drug and polymers first and then the ratios which give good formulations (physical evaluations) should be selected for the next phase of studies. Finally, only the selected ones should be studied in vivo. This holds true for other fields of research in one or more different ways. The key message is "Proceed step by step in a systematic way."

Sample analysis

While processing for analysis of samples, sampling should be done in proper way. Sample should be representative of the bulk. Sample may be defined as "   ". Samples should be taken in appropriate quantity and with right technique. The timing of sample should also be appropriate and preferably as per established guidelines, if any. For example for single point study the protocols of sample collection should be as per USFDA guidelines. For SR dosage form the timing of sample withdrawing should be as per the monograph of the drug in the pharmacopeias (IP or USP). The time difference between sampling and analysis should not be too great otherwise the results may get affected adversely. If the analysis is to be done after a major time lag then the samples should be properly packed in an airtight container and stored in required conditions like freezer, desiccator etc. If the samples are to be sent for analysis by post or by other means then their packaging should be able to sustain and bear the stress of transshipment (Refer Appendix 3: Directory of analytical service providers).

Data treatment and analysis

Most of the journals do not accept a research paper in which data are not treated statistically. Studies are performed in a way that readings can be taken to provide statistically significant means (Standard error of means). Data are generally taken in triplicate (n=3) or sometimes as n=5. Data should always elicit Standard error of means (SEM) and the values should be provided after the mean reading with $\pm$ sign (e.g. 2.45$\pm$ 0.024 mg).

The correlation between two set of data must be established and the correlation coefficient (R^2) must be calculated and presented in text. Equation of Line (in $Y=mX + C$ form) should be provided for linear curves.

Significance of data should be provided by performing a suitable statistical method like student' t test, F test, Analysis of variance (ANOVA), Chi square etc. For these statistical operations good texts of Biostatistics should be referred. You can also take the help of published articles and see the way of their presentation. These operations can be done manually as well as by the help of computers. By using MS-Excel these operations can be done by relatively very easily in a very short time. You must learn the use of MS excel for performing these statistical studies. Some special software like SPSS are also available for fitting the data and getting the statistical results.

For data analysis and interpretation the supervisor must be consulted. The supporting information and articles should be mentioned wherever you interpret the data and correlate the same with outcomes of other studies.

Sticking to time and work schedule

The most important component of research is following the time and work schedule. The performance of research work should be reviewed periodically for compliance with the PERT chart. In simple words do every work in predefined time and if delayed in a step, the time lapsed should be covered in the very next step. If we can cover more work in a particular step this is very nice as it may give as a bonus time in any unexpected delay in next tasks. The time delays may be of avoidable and unavoidable types. You can avoid the delays in which you and your lab work and conditions are the sole factor. On the other hand unavoidable delays include delay in getting the results of analysis from other institutes. The contingent plan should be ready for any type of avoidable delays and for some type of unavoidable delays also. Like if you have not got the sample analyzed in the expected time, take the information about the status, and follow up the institute in which the samples have been sent. In emergency, go to the institute directly and request for the analysis of samples on priority and get the results with you.

But you should not compromise the quality of work for meeting the deadlines always. Even if you do not give sufficient time to your binder (of thesis) the thesis shall not look professional. And this unfruitful saving of time shall pinch you always whenever you see the thesis in your life.

CHAPTER 13

Results and Discussion

Now you have got the results of all your studies. For simple experiments this is the finishing point of the exercise, but for the research work this is the part which adds the value to the work. Simply providing the results are just a cluster of observations. So to reach up to the fruitful conclusion it is utmost necessary to present the data in a comprehensive and pragmatic manner so that it becomes easy to discuss and draw the conclusion out of them. Compiling the results includes the following components.

Tabulation of results

The results should be tabulated whenever it is feasible. Even when the result of a parameter is not of more than one set, the results of this parameter should be grouped and tabulated with the result of the same parameter for other subjects. This may also be grouped and tabulated to observe any correlation or relevancy with other different or relevant parameter. A table should possess the following parts essentially.

1. Type: Tables should be of uniform type in the thesis. (Various types of tables can be found in MS Office tool bar of table).

2. Layout: Preferably should be in portrait (not in landscape)

3. Title: A brief, clear and easy to understand title

4. Column and Rows: Number of divisions and subdivisions of column or rows should not be confusing.

5. Heading: Heading of each column or row should be very brief and complete in all respect (unit of measurement etc.)

6. Footnote: Any extra information (p value, abbreviation etc.) for a particular set of data should be given in footnote, by providing asterisk or any other mark to the relevant data in the table. This is not compulsory to provide foot note to each table.

7. Grid lines: The grid lines should be clear enough to show the partitioning between column and rows. Sometimes hiding the gridlines make the table confusing.

In tables, unnecessary colors in column and rows should be avoided. You can directly paste any table from MS excel worksheet to MS word file also. This shall save your time.

Plotting graphs

Graphs should be plotted using MS excel worksheet. The Graphs may be of various types:

Pie Chart: When data can be shown in percent or parts the pie chart can be used. The pie chart is presentation of data in a circle (2D or 3D) to show the data or readings in percent or parts.

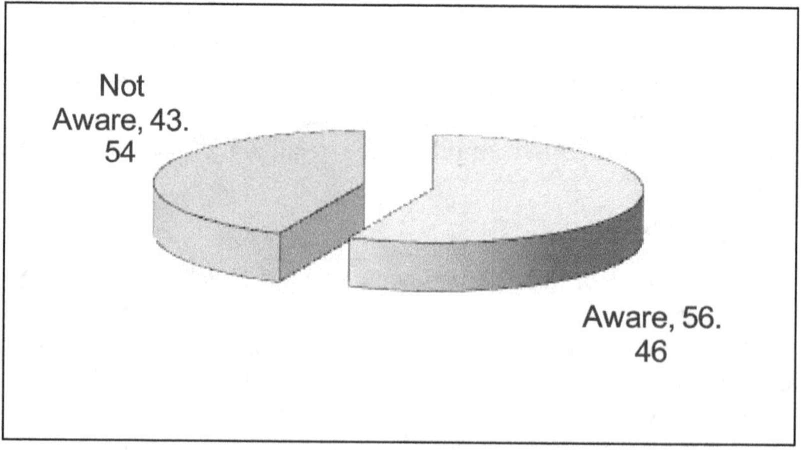

Fig. 1. Gender Distribution of Immunized Population (Pie Chart).

Bar diagram: The column form of data presentation is done in between X and Y axis. This is useful in giving the direct comparison between two set of observations with same set of variables. For example: Population living in different district of a state (Population in Y axis and District in X axis), Initiation time and completion time of hair growth by test standard and control (Time in Y axis, set of initiation time and completion time for test standard and control group of animals)

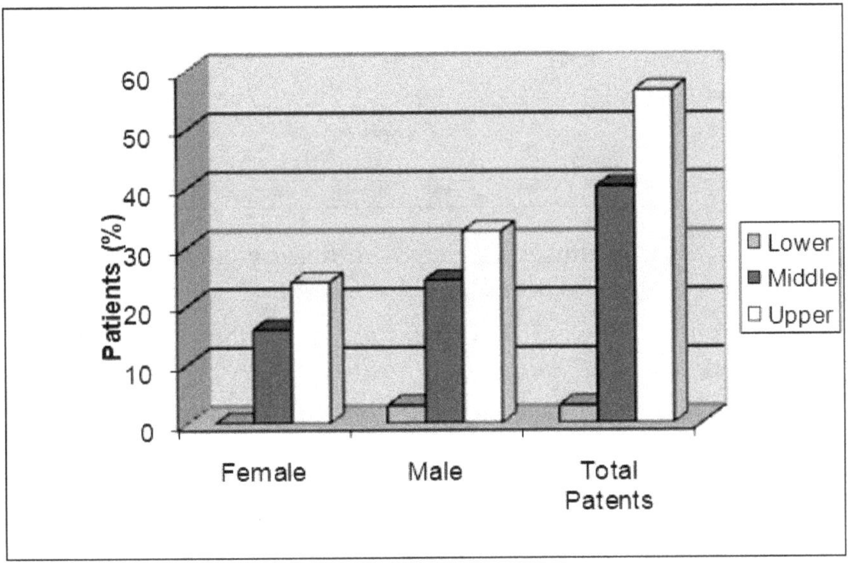

Fig. 2. Occurrence of Diabetes mellitus in different socioeconomic groups (Bar Diagram).

Line curve: This is the presentation of progression or change of a variable at different set of another variable. These are the most common chart used to show the growth of microbes with time, release of drug with time etc.

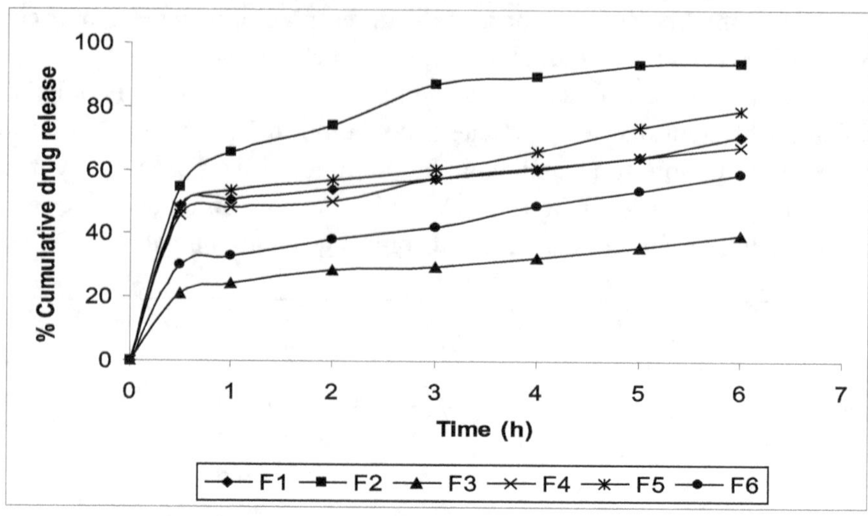

Fig. 3. *In vitro* drug release study of floating microspheres of Ofloxacin. (Line Curve).

A graph has the following component and all of these should be given due attention.

1. Data: Accurate data should be placed in worksheet in the right way.

2. Axis: X and Y axis should be taken with due care with the appropriate maximum and minimum values of scale (to give a right view to the graph). The major and minor units of scale should be according to the desired and full display of data.

3. Labeling: Axis should be labelled along with the unit of measurement.

4. Gridlines: X and or Y axis' gridlines may be shown if desired for certain purpose.

5. Legends: Legends should be clear, brief, and easy to identify. The colors or the sign of legend of a particular set of data should be unique in a single graph. The layout and positioning legends should be uniform for all graphs (i.e. Vertical layout and Bottom right positioning).

6. Error bars: Many high impact journals demand inclusion of error bars in each line curve and bar diagram. This can be done with the help of MS excel.

While pasting the graphs from excel to word sheet, you can either paste the graph as entire worksheet, or with link to work sheet or only as a curve with no link. If you paste the curve with entire worksheet, you can edit the graph from the word file itself. You do not need to go and search the desired worksheet in excel. However, if you opt for graph only paste option, then no one can access the data and edit the same in any case (from the word file).

Previous reports and references for explanation and discussion

Discussion is the most vital part of the research work. Without this part, none can draw any fruitful and concrete conclusion from the results. Discussion part should be dealt with an analytical way. The major work which should be done in this part should be as followed.

1. Put the results in the sequence in which you want to discuss.
2. Group the results of two or more set of studies which need establishment of any relation.
3. Take the results one by one.
4. Refer the related results of related work from the previous published research articles.
5. Report and mention the studies which support your results (i.e. have similar results).
6. Try to understand the reasoning and relationship of set of results.
7. Discuss the reasoning and relationship by taking the reference from previous studies and from your own experience (Supervisor's experience) and understanding.
8. Do not hesitate to report negative results. This may be highlighting any other parameters which other studies have not focused. Try to identify the reason.

CHAPTER 14

Empirical or Field Studies

Many studies are conducted in the form of field surveys. In these field or empirical studies the various information are gathered with the help of various tools like written or verbal questionnaires, interviews, opinion polls etc. from the target population or subjects. The national census is the largest kind of empirical study with a wide variety of objectives. The role of these studies are very important with respect to the research works pertaining to various subjects like management, commerce, economics, mass communication and social sciences. In the pharmaceutical sciences the research work of clinical pharmacy, pharmacy practice and hospital pharmacy are mainly utilize these studies for the research work.

Components of Empirical or field study

- Clear aim and SMART objectives

  From the origin of the idea to its subdivision into objectives is a very crucial and deciding task of a field study. The success of a field study depends on effective incubation of idea into feasible and practical plans.

For example if you want to know the feasibility of hepatitis B vaccination program in a local population, you need to know various things in a field study like how many persons are vaccinated in the local population (or representative local population), age distribution etc.

In a study by authors (Semalty et al., 2009) to focus on the status of awareness and Hepatitis B vaccination in the local population and to formulate the model plan to improve the awareness and vaccination status, the aim of the study was subdivided into following objectives:

1. To know the awareness about the disease among the local population (Hepatitis B)

2. To know the percentage of vaccination among local population

3. To focus the ratio of vaccination among male, female and children.

4. To correlate the relationship of literacy with percent vaccination among male and female.

5. To formulate the model plan to improve the awareness and vaccination status.

- Subject (selection and exclusion)

The subjects should be finalized based on various parameters as followed: weight, population, sex, age etc. If certain subjects with some specific properties are not needed or needed to be excluded then the exclusion criteria must be finalized. For clinical studies and health related surveys the exclusion criteria may be based on various parameters of subjects like the habits (smoking, drinking etc.), sex (male, female), physiological or pathophysiological status (e.g. pregnancy, hypertensive patients), age (infants, older people).

- Study Area (geographical, epidemiological, literacy, economy etc.)

The study area should be selected based on aim and objectives. The feasibility to execute the program in a study area should be finalized based on information related to geographical, epidemiological, literacy and economy of the population. In the earlier discussed study (Semalty et al 2009) we selected the two major governmental hospitals of the local area and collected the required data from the population (patients, their relatives, health workers, and others) coming into the hospitals for 15 days.

- Tool of the study (questionnaire, interview, mail/postal survey etc.)

  The selection of tool of the study should be made intelligently based on literacy level of the subjects, economy of the execution of study, and quality/effectiveness of the data. The tools may be any of the following

  - ➢ Questionnaire: A well designed and validated set of open/close ended questions framed in local language.

  - ➢ Interviews: Flexible number and nature of questioned can be designed which may be helpful in deducing the results.

  - ➢ Postal and email surveys: Postal and electronic mails may also be used to get the required information or data.

- Execution of study

  After planning the study with respect to subject, study area and tools of study, the vital part is execution. A well designed study can be executed relatively with greater ease and accuracy. The use of the tools of the study whether conducting questionnaire based or interview based or any other way it should be done in taking due consideration of comfort level of responder. The questionnaire must not be used in the form of brushfire of questions. The care should be taken in questioning more private or religious issues. The timing of the study should be well suited to responders. The natural and original data collection should be emphasized. If the data is being collected by a team, the team leader should take the follow up of the study conduction.

- Collecting/compiling data

  When you have got the raw data compile the same to give the same a shape of meaningful and easy to interpret manner. The compilation of data may be in tabular form or chart form. Exclude the data about which you are not sure. The data should be categorized with respect to cater the objectives of the study. The compilation of data should be done in such a way that it may easily be treated statistically.

- Data treatment

  In the field study this is the statistics which make the compilation of data meaningful. The data are treated statistically using suitable methods. The help of computer software like SPSS may be taken to get the concluding remark. The significance of data must be checked and reported properly. Moreover, the acceptance criteria, degree of freedom etc should be clearly mentioned. Use the established methods like chi square, F test, ANOVA depending upon the requirement of the data and the study. Plot relevant curves, diagram etc to visualize the results.

- Discussion and Reaching objectives

Now report the results of the study clearly and try to discuss it by taking the help of previous related study. Justify your results, defend any negative result (if you have the rational answer) and report if any unexpected results are seen. Conclude the results stating the constraints of the study.

CHAPTER 15

Report Writing

Writing a scientific report is a science as well as an art. You can make an average work very noticeable while on the other hand even if you have done a path breaking piece of work, it would be a trash if not reported and presented effectively. So don't take a sigh of relief after executing the study and compiling the data. Now the time comes to show your work in a way that elicits your hard work and which shows your vital contribution in the field of the study. The report writing has various components which must be taken seriously to give the report a professional and scientific look. In the present chapter we shall discuss all the components of report writing one by one.

(a) Planning of chapters

First of all an outline of the thesis must be prepared. This should begin with the planning of chapters to be included in the report. In general all the science projects and thesis are planned with following sequence of chapters.

1. Introduction
2. Literature review

3. Material and Methods
4. Results and discussion
5. Conclusion
6. References/bibliography
7. Appendices

However the chapters may be planned according to our need or as mentioned or planned in the synopsis. You can have a common or different material & methods and Results & Discussion chapter depending on the nature and number of the study subjects. For example if you have studied the three plants with respect to their antidiabetic activity plan three separate chapters for result and discussion. Pharmaceutics researchers can split the chapters in formulation & evaluation and results & discussion. The central idea is the planning of chapters should be self explanatory, complimentary to the objective of the study and easy to review.

(b) Commencing the writing with Introduction

Introduce the topic effectively and give the historical background of the study area and then of the specific study (of drug or plant etc.). Clarify the origin of the idea.

Naringenin is a flavonoid specific to citrus fruits and possesses anti-inflammatory, anticarcinogenic, and antitumor effects. But due to a lower half-life and rapid clearance from the body, frequent administration of the molecule is required. To improve the bioavailability and prolong its duration in body system, its phospholipid complexes were prepared by a simple and reproducible method. – Semalty et al. 2010

As various plant parts especially seeds have been reported to be used externally for various skin diseases, it was hypothesized it might have antimicrobial activity also. Therefore the present study was performed to evaluate the antibacterial and antifungal activity of flowers and pods of P. pinnata. - Kumar et al. 2010

Also state major approaches so far carried to cater the problem you have identified. Draw the attention towards the need of the study, rationality, and its expected outcome. Do not unnecessarily increase the length of introduction part. Too lengthy introduction lose their rhythm and focusing. In general you can plan an introduction of 10-20 pages (12 font, double space, times new roman)

(c) Planning of a good literature survey with analytical preview

Literature review should ideally be written in parallel to your execution part. This shall give you the valuable inputs to identify problems, selecting the proper formulation/plan of work or resolving the problem arising in execution. As we have earlier mentioned that it is better to prepare a review paper on the study area and get published. It would have two potential advantages 1) Inclusion of a paper in the thesis increases its acceptability and rationality. 2) The literature review chapter is just ready with almost zero defects. During the preparation of manuscript of a paper you have already checked it several times and thereafter rest of the work is done by the peer reviewing process itself.

The literature review may be subdivided or made convergent from broad to specific area of study. The specific citation should be current and be presented in chronological order (2010, 2009 then 2008 and so on). Do not include very old references until they are inevitable to mention. You can take the flow of literature review to the state of the art, current and advanced work slowly so that the rhythm of the chapter is not lost. You should not simply paste the abbreviated version of abstract of the studies rather the studies should be analytically reviewed with respect to your study's need. The tone should be unbiased. Avoid using the words "They did the study….., he concluded….., he found". Write in passive voice to avoid these words. Like in place of writing "he concluded that…" you should write "it was concluded that".

You can split the review as per your need. For example if you are doing the work on antidiabetic activity of some plants then plan the review as followed: 1) Review of diabetes and its current treatment and their drawbacks 2) Herbal antidiabetics 3) Plant reviews (covered with related and other activities)

(d) Main research/ experimental work: Procedure, observations, and presentation of data

In this part, describe the methodology/ procedures/ protocol, observations, and results of your study. This section is variously called Experimental/Methods or Materials and Methods. This is the heart of a thesis as well as of a research paper.

Function: In this section you explain *clearly* how you carried out your study in the following *general* structure and organization (details follow below):

You should begin with details of materials. The source of the chemical, reagents, polymers and drugs be mentioned clearly under the heading if materials. Methods should be clearly described with each specifications and experimental conditions. Whenever discussed for the first time, equipment's model, make and country should be mentioned within the brackets after its name like *"In vitro dissolution studies for drug complex as well as plain drug were performed in triplicate in a USP XXIII six station dissolution test apparatus (Veego Model No. 6DR, India) at 100 rpm and at 37 ^0C".*

- the subjects used (plant, animal, human, etc.) and their pre-experiment handling and care, and when and where the study was carried out (if location and time are important factors);

- if a field study, a description of the study site, including the physical and biological features, and precise location;

- the experimental OR sampling design (i.e., how the experiment or study was structured. For example, controls, treatments, the variable(s) measured, how many samples were collected, replication, etc.);

- the protocol for collecting data, i.e., how the experimental procedures were carried out, and,

- how the data were analyzed (statistical procedures used).

Organize your presentation so your reader will understand the logical flow of the experiment(s); subheadings work well for this purpose. Each experiment or procedure should be presented as a unit, even if it was broken up over time. In general, provide enough quantitative detail (how much, how long, when, etc.) about your experimental protocol such that other scientists could reproduce your experiments. You should also indicate the **statistical procedures** used to analyze your results, including the probability level at which you determined significance (usually at 0.05 probability).

Style: The style in this section should read as if you were verbally describing the conduct of the experiment. You may use the active voice to a certain extent, although this section requires more use of third person, passive constructions than others. Avoid use of the first person in this section. Remember to use the past tense throughout. The Methods section *is not* a step-by-step, directive, protocol as you might see in your lab manual.

Describe the organism(s) used in the study. This includes giving the *source* (supplier or *where* and *how* collected), *size, how they were handled* before the experiment, what they were fed, etc. In genetics studies include the strains or genetic stocks used.

Describe the site where your field study was conducted. The description must include both *physical* and *biological* characteristics of the site pertinent to the study aims. Include the date(s) of the study (e.g., 10-15 April 1994) and the exact location of the study area.

Describe your experimental design clearly. Be sure to include the *hypotheses* you tested, *controls, treatments, variables* measured, how many *replicates* you had, what you measured, what form the *data* take, etc. Always identify treatments by the variable or treatment name, NOT by an ambiguous, generic name or number (e.g., use "2.5% saline" rather than "test 1".) If your paper contain more than one experiment or tests use subheadings to organize your presentation. A general experimental design worksheet is available to help plan your experiments in the core courses.

Describe the protocol for your study in sufficient detail that other scientists could repeat your work to verify your findings. Foremost in your description should be the "quantitative" aspects of your study - the masses, volumes, incubation times, concentrations, etc., that another scientist needs to duplicate your experiment. When using standard lab or field methods and instrumentation, it is not always necessary to explain the procedures (e.g., serial dilution) or equipment used (e.g., autopipette) since other scientists will likely be familiar with them already. You may want to identify certain types of equipment by brand or category (e.g., ultracentrifuge vs. prep centrifuge). It is appropriate to give the source for reagents used parenthetically, e.g., "....poly-l-Lysine (Sigma #1309)." When using a method described in another published source, you can save time and words by referring to it and providing the relevant citation to the source. Always make sure to describe any modifications you have made of a standard or published method.

Describe how the data were summarized and analyzed. Here you will indicate what types of data summaries and analyses were employed to answer each of the questions or hypotheses tested.

The information should include:

- how the data were summarized (Means, percent, etc) and how you are reporting measures of variability (SD,SEM, etc)

- data transformation (e.g., to normalize or equalize variances)

- statistical tests used with reference to the questions they address, e.g.,

   "A Paired t-test was used to compare mean flight duration before and after applying stabilizers to the glider's wings."

   "One way ANOVA was used to compare mean weight gain in weight-matched calves fed the three different rations."

- any other numerical or graphical techniques used to analyze the data

   Here is some additional advice on problems common to new scientific writers.

Problem*: The Methods section is prone to being wordy or overly detailed.*

- *Avoid repeatedly using a single sentence to relate a single action*; this results in very lengthy, wordy passages. A related sequence of actions can be combined into one sentence to improve clarity and readability:

Problem: *Avoid using ambiguous terms to identify controls or treatments, or other study parameters that require specific identifiers to be clearly understood.* Designators such as Tube 1, Tube 2, or Site 1 and Site 2 are completely meaningless out of context and difficult to follow in context.

The data should be presented in a simple and easy to understand way. Do not make the simple things complex. If some result can be stated in a single sentence do not attempt the tabular or other presentation of the same. It is not necessary to give each raw data in the thesis (Ph D). However, sometimes a supervisor may ask to incorporate all the triplicate readings to be mentioned in M. Pharm or other post graduate dissertation work. In general, the average readings followed by ± SEM (standard error of means or standard deviation) are shown in tabular forms. The significant data or the insignificant data must be marked in the table with single or double asterisk (*, **). The graphs plotted should be self explanatory. The legends (signs referring to a particular series in the graph) should be clear, visible, and well illustrated or mentioned either within the graph or in the title of the graph. Check whether the X and Y axis lines are of good weight or not. The axis lines sometimes are not visible fully in printouts. So increase their weights from excel sheet. The numbers in axes should be of uniform font and size throughout the thesis. The size of the graph should also be made uniform. Graph and tables should be placed as close to as the place in which those are being discussed first time. Their placement should not affect the rhythm of language also. Preferable graph and tables should be in portrait layout. The landscape figures are generally typical to see. So make the things easier to read.

(e)   Results

This is the most important part of the thesis. Its upon to you whether you want to give all the results first and then discussing the same. Or alternatively you can write the results and discussion simultaneously. Ultimately you should be in position to reach the aim and objectives of the study. No question should be unanswered.

The result part is probably the easiest to write, as it is a compilation of facts and observations. This section provides the evidence that leads to the answers of the study to the question you posed at the start. The reader should be guided to these findings by using the text of the results along with a judicious use of tables and illustrations. Start the section with what you have did in the study (in brief like In the present experiment naringenin–phospholipid complex were prepared by a simple and reproducible method with the aim to improving the bioavailability of naringenin.) Then take the results of experiments one by one.

Narrative is a good style but avoid terms like 'majority, 'most of the patients', 'in some cases', 'significantly greater than etc. Follow a sequence, do not jump from one group of animals to another and then back to the first. All the groups must be accounted for in Results. If some results are paradoxical let them state as such. You should not even afraid of reporting the negative results. Even the negative results contribute to research and development. Never ever manipulate the data for making them more effective and for exaggerating the beneficial effects or positive results. An expert reviewer can easily trace the manipulations and this may result in bad consequences. Even a small manipulation can make your whole work questionable and unreliable.

(f)   Discussion

It is usually a good idea to begin this section by giving the answer to the question you set out with.

- Take the results one by one and discuss them. Support your result or conclusion with previous work done. Mention the studies which showed the similar results in some other drug/plant/system etc. Compare this data with other published information and bring out the similarities and conflicts, if any. You may find crucial information in someone else's study that helps you interpret your own data, or perhaps you will be able to reinterpret others' findings considering yours. In either case you should discuss reasons for similarities and differences between yours and others' findings. Consider how the results of other studies may be combined with yours to derive a new or perhaps better substantiated understanding of the problem. Be sure to state the conclusions that can be drawn from your results considering these considerations.

- You should not **introduce new results (from your study) in the Discussion.**

- Try to understand the mechanism of changes in results with different batches or formulations or plants. Give the statement or expression of probable relation and cause of observed trend in results. Analytically review the statistical treatment of data and justify the genuineness, originality, correlation, and trends shown by the data in the results.

- Interpretation of your results includes discussing how your results modify and fit in with what we previously understood about the problem. Review the literature again currently. After completing the experiments you will have much greater insight into the subject, and by going through some of the literature again, information that seemed trivial before, or was overlooked, may tie something together and therefore prove very important to your own interpretation. Be sure to cite the works that you refer to.

In research papers as well as in the thesis most of the reviewers give the prime attention to this part of the paper in the process of reviewing.

(g) Conclusion

In some cases the conclusion can be given at the end of results and discussion. But alternatively a one page conclusion can be givens separately. You should just mention the conclusion in three stanza. First: dealing with aim and need of the study; Second: dealing with the experiment done and Last with result (sometimes the future or further studies needed to be done are added).

(h) References

References should be cited in the text in a particular uniform way. There may be several ways of citing the references in text.

......XX [5–7]; .....XX [5–7]; .....XX 5–7 ; ...XX (Semalty et al., 2010).

You can adapt any one and follow it uniformly. In case you are adapting the last type the references should be given alphabetically in the reference section.

The reference writing should also be uniform.

- **Journal Article**

    Type 1:

    Franklin M, Estabrook R. On the inhibitory action of mersalyl on microsomal drug oxidation: A rigid organization of the electron transport chain. Arch. Biochem. 1971;143:318-329.

    Type 2:

    Saito Y, Jinno K (2002) Anal Bioanal Chem 373:325–331.

    Type 3:

    P. Ahlin, J. Kristl and J. Smid-Korbar, Optimisation of procedure parameters and physical stability of solid lipid nanoparticles in dispersions, *Acta Pharm.* 48 (1998) 259-267.

Book

Entire book

Type 1:

Macomber R. A Complete Introduction to Modern NMR Spectroscopy. New York: John Wiley & Sons; 1998.

Type 2:

Manz A, Becker H (1999) (eds) Microsystem technology in chemistry and life sciences. Springer, Berlin Heidelberg NewYork

Type 3:

E. Mutchler and H. Derendorf, *Drug Actions, Basic Principles and Therapeutic Aspects,* Medpharm Scientific Publishers, Stuttgart 1995, pp. 16-26.

Chapter in a book

Levy G. The case for preclinical pharmacodynamics. In: Yacobi A, Skelly J, Shah V, Benet L, eds. Integration of Pharmacokinetics, Pharmacodynamics, and Toxicokinetics in Rational Drug Development, New York: Plenum Press, 1993;7-13.

Example for patent reference:

H. P. Wang, O. Lee and C. T. Fan, *Preparation of Gemfibrozil Analogs as Anticholinergic Compounds,* U.S. Pat. 5,530,145, 25 Jun 1996; ref. *Chem. Abstr.* 125 (1996) 142277u.

Thesis or Dissertation

Thorn MD. *A Comparative Review of the Statistical and Research Quality of the Medical and Pharmacy Literature* [masters thesis]. Chapel Hill: University of North Carolina, 1982.

Reference to a Web Site. For references to journals, e-magazines, or other publications on the Internet, state the names of the authors, title of the article, publication title, and volume and publication date in the same format as you would for a journal reference. For references to other information, give the title of the web page, followed by the name of the organization or web site that published the information. For all references to online material, the author should include "Available at:" followed by the uniform resource locator (URL) for the page of the web site referenced (eg, www.hcfa.gov/stats.htm), followed by a period. Finally, write "Accessed" followed by the month, day, and year on which the information was obtained from the site, followed by a period.

Example:

Healthy People 2010, Office of Disease Prevention and Health Promotion, U.S. Department of Health and Human Services. Available at: http://health.gov/healthypeople. Accessed January 20, 2002.

Unpublished Works. References to unpublished material such as articles or abstracts presented at professional meetings but not published, provide the name of the meeting where the article was presented.

Articles in Press. For references to information in books or articles that are currently in press, provide all the available information for the reference. In place of page numberS, designate that the publication is "in press."

Example:

Adamcik B, Hurley S, Erramouspe J. Assessment of pharmacy students' critical thinking and problem-solving abilities. *Am J Pharm Educ.* 1996;60:in press.

So any one style may be adopted in a thesis. In chemistry thesis generally the title of the article is avoided to make the referencing easy. For example: S. L. Bartley, K. R. Dunbar, *Angew. Chem.* **1991**, *103*, 447-450.

In the authors opinion references should generally be given in the same way as the prescribed by the journal in which you are aiming to publish the research paper coming out of the work. This would save the time in preparing the manuscript. The accuracy of references should be taken with extra care. Nowadays software are available to check the accuracy of the references.

(i) Summary

In Ph D thesis you are required to submit the summary of the work in the same number as that of the thesis. Plan chapter wise summary or abstract and compile them. Each chapter's summary should state the contents or the matter discussed in the particular chapter. Never ever take the summary lightly. Many a times the thesis reviewer make the summary as the basis of the evaluation. The length of the summary should be around 8 to 12 pages depending upon the number of chapters. Each chapters summary should neither be too brief nor too lengthy. At least, important results must be mentioned (as you provide in preparing the abstract of a paper).

(j) Style and Typesetting common uses of computers

The typesetting is the most tedious task for the persons who are not friendly with computers. However, this work can be got done by professional typesetters but we strongly recommend that you do it yourself. In this way you shall maintain the accuracy, rhythm, and command over your work. Generally there are following phases of typesetting.

1. **Setting margins:** Consult you binder about the space he need in the margins. This shall be dependent upon the type of binding. In general the left margin should be liberal and sufficient enough to provide the full view and opening of the pages. The top bottom and right margins should also be sufficient to provide the space for cutting and leveling the pages during binding. If margins are not proper even a good thesis looks odd.

2. **Font:** Font size should be optimum. Many a times, Universities provide the guidelines regarding the writing the thesis. In those cases the guidelines should be strictly followed. In general a font size of 12 (Times New Roman) in double spacing is kept in the thesis. However font size 13 can also be tried.

3. **Headings and subheadings:** Headings should be clear, brief, and complimentary to the rhythm of the text. The headings and subheadings should look different. For this you can put the headings in title case with Upper case and/ or bold letters, Subheadings in sentence case, Bold/normal faced and sub-subheadings in sentence case, normal face, italics. The headings level can also be done with numbers like 1. Heading; 1.1 subheading; 1.1.1 sub-subheading and so on.

4. **Chapter Titles:** The title of chapters may be given in a separate page in mono or color. It may also be given before the introduction part of the chapter. But in that case the font size must be higher than headings (generally 18 to 24 in Bold and upper/ title case.

5. **Header and Footer:** Header may be the name of chapter and the footer may be the name of the institute. They should be in small font (generally 10 or 11), Title case, bold/normal face, and italics. The spelling mistakes must be avoided because it is more likely to draw the attention and hence may leave a bad impression.

6. **Paragraph setting:** Paragraphs should be given liberal before and after space (Generally 6 or 12). A new heading or a new para should start in a new page, if possible.

7. **Table and Figures:** See the look of tables and figures and finalize their position. Many a times Figure and table sizes are left disproportionate and non-uniform. Place the tables and

figures as near as possible to their citation. Try to put to two figures in a single page if they are being discussed together. In that case do not insert the running text in that page. The figures should be of the size which allows clear presentation of results. But they should not be too large also. It is a wrong habit to put a large, single figure in a single page to enhance the number of pages.

8. **Equations and special characters:** Give attention to presentation of equations. Its better to write the equations in Microsoft equation (a function in MS Word). The special characters like micron (μ), beta (β), Rho (ρ), gamma (γ) etc. should be checked specially for their accurate presentation. Sometime they get changed automatically upon pasting from a pdf file to word file.

(k) Cover or Title Page

The cover or title page is generally standard for a particular University. So refer any previous years' (or current) thesis, put all the required things (title, your name and enrollment number, subject, Logo of University, year of submission, Supervisor's name and the name of the institution). Give utmost attention to the title. It must be matched word to word with the title mentioned in your registration letter. Even addition or deletion of simply "a", "the" or "some" may lead to problem in submission. If it happens you have to unbound all the thesis again, get the changes and resubmit. This shall delay the submission only.

(l) Auxiliary parts of reports (Acknowledgement, Index, appendixes etc.)

When you have prepared the whole text of your thesis or project, plan auxiliary parts of the same. These are not very much important part but they add the value to the work. In acknowledgement (placed after the supervisor's certificate) acknowledge each one who have helped you or extended the technical, nontechnical, or moral support. This is your personal page so you have the liberty to thank anyone. Index (placed after acknowledgement) should be provided either exhaustively sothat each heading discussed are mentioned with the concerned page number or simply a gross indexing with the chapters name and page numbers. Its all upto you or on prescribed guidelines (if any). Appendixes (placed at the end of the thesis) can be given for list of publications, list of abbreviations, material and their source, equipment, and their source etc.

(m) Final checking and proofreading

Get the print out and check the thesis finally and proofread the same. Mark the changes and correct them. When you are fully satisfied take another printout, bind it in spiral and get it checked from your supervisor. When the supervisors has checked the same take a final print in bond paper (85 or 120 gsm) and again get it checked by the supervisor. If the final prints are okay you can go ahead for other copies of the same. Do not forget to take the letterhead of supervisor, print the supervisor's certificate or any other prescribed format, insert the same in each copy and then give the same to binder.

(n) Binding and submission

Select a good binder based on his previous work. Give the required details like number of copies of thesis and summary, type of binding, Cover/front page and its color or style, position of transparencies (before figures and chapter names), time required, and your contact number. Do not forget to take the contact number of binder and follow up the progress of work. Always very carefully proofread the front page designed by him. Give him the instructions if you want the front page as the embossed one. However, nowadays computer designed cover page is more popular. The type of binding material and its color should also be confirmed and informed. Once the thesis and summary copies are ready check them again for completeness or for any mistake. Now sign the each copy of the thesis with a good pen and then get the sign of your supervisor. Then proceed for final submission of the thesis in the University. All university demand the submission of sift copy of the thesis in CD. So write the CD with the complete thesis, label the same with the title of thesis, year, subject, your name and roll number. Put the CD in unit plastic CD box or CD mailer and submit the same with the hard copies. Never forget to take the submission certificate immediately after the submission. Once you have got the submission certificate you can take a sigh of relief and enjoy.

(o) Supervisor' role

A good supervisor is more than a boon. It is the supervisor who can make a difference in your research work. A supervisor plays a very vital role. Supervisor helps in planning and designing of the work. He or she takes you out of the problem. A constant supervision by supervisor in execution phase avoids any blunders. This is the duty of the student to get in close touch with his or her supervisor. As supervisor may be busy in his or her various other academic duties, the suitable time slot should be requested from him by the student. Daily, weekly, fortnightly, or monthly reporting should be done. The reporting should be in complete form. You should carry all the raw and processed data to show the supervisor. Any serious problem must be discussed with supervisor after a good homework. The routine reports which are to be sent in the University should be discussed, checked, and approved by the supervisor. No change in work should be made without the consent of the supervisor.

When completing your work each component of thesis should be planned and designed as per supervisor's instructions. Give the contents of the thesis chapter by chapter for checking. If he says you should be present during the checking so that you may know the changes or clarification he wants. When you have received the checked chapter, then give him the next one and meanwhile make the changes in previous chapter as per supervisor's comments. Do not force your supervisor to check the chapters in hurry. This shall lower the quality of evaluation.

(p) Planning and writing a research paper

In the new regulations (2009) of submission Ph D thesis, the thesis must be submitted along with at least one published research paper in a referred (peer reviewed) journal. So roll your sleeves and plan a research paper. Planning a research paper should begin just after the end of you execution phase. Plan the paper early so that you get it published by the time of your thesis submission. It is easy to write a thesis or dissertation report but it is too tough to get it published in a reputed journal. In this work you should take the guidance of your supervisor. Plan a paper, search a good and relevant journal, see the authors' instructions, draft the manuscript accordingly, check it yourself and then give the same to your supervisor for checking and then submit on line or off line. Prefer the journal who give the decisions in short time and who are having the web based manuscript submission process. This saves the time and efforts. When you receive the comment of reviewers, read them very carefully, discuss with the supervisor and then modify the manuscript accordingly. In submitting the revised manuscript, address the each individual comment. Revise the manuscript as early as possible (after getting the comments) with full attention and then resubmit the revised version. If you do not get the answer in time give the reminder to the editor. When your paper is accepted a copyright form is sent to you. Fill it, declare any funding or grant received, association with a company, sign it, scan it and then submit the sift copy (in web based system). Then you are provided the galley proof of your article. See the pdf file of the paper with full attention. Submit the correction and approve the proof (on line or offline). In a due course of time you will get the reprints of the article (in ahead of print form without pagination). Some journals provide the reprints only when they are published in the print version. The details of writing a research paper shall be discussed in the next chapter.

CHAPTER 16

Presentation of Work

Once you have got the date of your Ph D viva you start losing your nerves. Simply because you have not faced any exam after your postgraduation. Do not be afraid of presenting the hard work you have done all through your Ph D tenure. Be confident of yourself and start preparing. Firstly prepare the power point presentation of your work under the following heads or according to your chapters. For a Ph D viva the slides may be 50 to even 80 but for PG projects they may be less (upto 40-50). The depth of the work determines the number of slides. Basically the slides should be minimized up to that extent to which they can easily and effectively be understood. Take the contents from your thesis and start preparing the slides as shown in the table ahead. Do not use more colorful and animated slides. The presentation slides should be simple and effective. Try to be brief in mentioning the text. When showing methods' slides just enumerate the methods in the slide and explain each method one by one during presentation. It is better to take the printout of the prepared slides and thoroughly check the same for any spelling and other kind of mistakes. Make the slides full proof. Even a very simple mistake looks awkward in the presentation. The attention drawn by a mistake during the presentation may lose your flow of presentation and your confidence. Also prepare the verbatim detailing of each individual slide and read it again and again and grasp the same. Get the slides as well as the detailing checked from you supervisor.

Table Preparation of power point slides for Ph D viva or presentation.

Name of section	Contents	Number of slides	Remarks
Title	Study title, names of student, supervisor, and the institute	01	Clear introduction of title
Introduction	Historical background, need of study	02-03	Establish rationality and need of the work
Literature review	Brief one or two lined introduction of major studies of literature review	04-05	Show the important work and their results
Aim of the study	Need, hypothesis, objectives	01-02	Establish rationality of the work
Materials and methods	Study materials and method details	02-04	Introduce study protocol and Methodology
Results	Processed and refined results	20-50	Tables and Figures only
Discussion	Mention the relation/ conflict with previous studies	10-15	Justify, interpret, and explain results
Conclusion	Concluding remark	01-02	Final answer to the study problem
Acknowledgements	Thanksgiving to guide, any grant, fellow researchers, staff, and others.	01	Show gratitude to all contributors and well wishers
References	Important references	01-02	Supporting references
Publications	List the publications out of the work	01-02	Even accepted papers can also be shown.
Thanks	-	01	Thanks and invite the questions

Prepare for defending probable questions

After preparing the slides, make a list of probable questions that may be asked by the examiner or anyone else. Also show the whole presentation to your fellow researcher and ask them about the probable questions. Also consult the supervisor. Ask about the probable question and then about the preparation of answers of the same. The questions should be heard attentively and then answered according to your understanding. If you do not know any answer simply say so. Do not be afraid of failure in addressing the questions asked by the examiner and the audience. Start with a smile and end with a smile. After addressing the questions again say thank to all and leave.

Components of effective scientific presentation

- **Command over the subject:** A scientific presentation always needs a good command over the subject or the topic. As you might not be touching every aspect of the topic but you should know about the related things. For this you must have an idea about the audience regarding their interests and familiarity with your topic. Their expectation regarding the presentation of either data or concept or both should be taken care of in preparing the slides. But you should always remember that a presentation is different than a paper. So don't try to cover everything. However in presentation of Ph D work you must prepare to show each and every data, but do not go into the detail until asked.

- **Command over the language:** Once you have gone through the verbatim detailing of speech, concentrate on you language in tune with your slides. Do not read the presentation. Practice the presentation so that you can speak from bullet points. The text should be a cue for the presenter rather than the full message for the audience.

- **Simple and effective designing of power point slides:** As we have mentioned earlier also that the slides should be simple and as brief as possible (in number as well as the quantity of text in a single slide). Do not use a lot of animation and special effects. In scientific presentations all these things look like gimmick and nothing else. Stick to plain backgrounds. Fancy formats are more appropriate for business presentations. Do not use a lot of colors, or wrong combination of colors like red green combinations and combinations of two light or two dark colors etc. Dark letters on a light background or vice versa should be chosen. Do not put a lot of text and figures in a single slide. Give only 3 to 4 lines in a slide. Leave empty space in each slide. Make the tables and figure simple and self explanatory. Choose a font style that your audience can read from a distance. Keep your text simple by using bullet points or short sentences. At last never forget to check the spelling and grammar.

- **Confidence:** To boost your confidence and enhance your presentation, you need to have enough preparation particularly your speech improvisation, as the way of gaining good rapport from your audience. Rehearse and practice a lot, until you are thorough with you verbatim detailing. Even the well known speakers rehearse well before the presentation. See your timing and your smooth transition from slides to slides. All these shall make you confident of your presentation.

- **Connectivity with audience:** Never ever lose the connectivity with you audience. It happens when you are not aware of the content exactly and you start reading the slide or you start writing an equation or drawing a figure on board. Even if you are writing the communication should not be paused. You should maintain the eye contact with you audience. If audience is more you can divide them in some small pockets and see in well balanced proportion during your entire presentation. By this you are giving importance to every member in audience. In quassi-scientific or non scientific presentation speaker may poke a joke, tell a story to get back your audience's attention. However it is still possible with the scientific presentation but the timing of putting the humor in your presentation is very important. Native speakers can successfully incorporate jokes into their presentations. However, it has been found that non-native speakers often cannot. A joke usually requires timing or pronunciation skills that a non-native speaker does not have. Also different cultures can be offended by jokes that we might find funny.

By ensuring that your script follows good storytelling conventions you can ensure the connectivity. You should give the script a beginning, middle, and end; have a clear arc that builds towards some sort of climax; make your audience appreciate each slide but be anxious to find out what is next; and when possible, always leave them wanting more. The basic aim is to attract and maintain the attention and interest of audience throughout the presentation.

What you are discussing should only be visible on the slide at a particular moment. Otherwise the audience may keep on reading and losing attention out of the point you are discussing. You should give the information and present it in a natural, systematic and in a rhythmic way.

In other than Ph D viva, every effort should be made to increase the involvement of your audience. You can do this by asking well thought out, appropriate questions. Do not think you should be a talking head right through your presentations. Why are you doing all the heavy lifting? Think of an attention grabbing question you could ask at the start and questions you could ask right through the presentation. This gets people thinking, lifts the energy in the room, and basically people hear some voices besides yours… which might be good thing!

- **Start and the end:** Start with a smile and end with a smile. Starter may be a formal hello followed by you introduction. May a times, a short story telling makes an environment. It depends all on your knowledge about the audience. So its better to come early know the audience and also ensure the proper working of you computers, your slides and other things which you are going to use in the presentation. Make yourself comfortable and then start. You also may chose to start without power point slides already opened and put a question before the audience as a starter. The question should be relevant and create the interest in the presentation. Like: *"Hope all you take a few mg of active drug in tablet or pill form of synthetic drugs and on the other hand a few 100 or 200 grams of herbal drugs. But, can the herbal drugs be given in the small quantities like tablets with same effectiveness as that of modern drugs?"* And for the same presentation the relevant end of the presentation may be *"YES, WE CAN!"*. The end may have any quote, some pictures etc. For scientific studies involving the animal tests the photographs of a group of albino rats with thanks may be a good end. You can put your creativeness in ending the conversation.

- **Communication skill (verbal):** You must communicate your message effectively. The communication skill needed to deliver an effective presentation is a nice blend of a good script, stories, figures, humors, and your ability to make the topic interested so that the audience remain connected. You should write a nice script and rehearse it well so that your slides are self explanatory and on the same time you should be able to illustrate and expand your idea to your audience effectively. You should know what to say and when to say, how to say and how to visualize it very precisely. You should always know when presenting which slide is coming up next. It sounds very powerful when you say "On the next slide [Click] you will see…", rather than a period of confusion when the next slide appears. In the beginning you must have an outline to follow in the whole presentation.

Correct pronunciation is important if one is to be understood correctly. Incorrect pronunciation is perhaps the first cause of communication breakdown. Always make sure you know how to correctly pronounce at least the key technical words or words that you repeat repeatedly in your speech.

Do not speak as if you are singing a lullaby. The voice, or more precisely the qualities of the voice should is a powerful tool of n effective presentation. The voce qualities include clarity, loudness, speed (fast or slow), variety, pitch (high or low), silent moments or pauses. The voice can be used to differentiate between a plain statement to a punch line (or key idea). The voice creates atmosphere. Its all depend on your quality of voice and with the same you can make the presentation effective, monotonous or help the audience to sleep!

- **Body language and Gestures:** Body language and gestures constitute the nonverbal communication skill. Body language should never be under estimated about its impact. We all believe in first impression and that is always nonverbal (body language and gesture). In each type of communication the nonverbal component play a major role. It is a visual and natural part of communication which is used to clarify meaning, to vent nervousness, to maintain interest and to emphasize.

Simply you should be natural and relaxed. You should stand tall, look confident, maintain eye contact with your audience and smile throughout the presentation. Your facial expressions should be natural and friendly. Use your hands properly during the presentation. Do not point the audience, welcome any question by open hands, do not fold the hands. While one hand in a pocket gives a very relaxed pose (and shows your confidence)but both hands in pockets looks too casual or awkward and should be avoided.

If you are using a podium, stand back a little so that you do not bend your head to read your text. Keep your arms by your sides but bend them from the elbow to gesture. Use body movements effectively. Use natural, conversational gestures. Move around, but between your key points. Do not do unnecessary or awkward body movements like scratching your nose, jiggling things in your pocket, or shuffling from foot to foot.

Check list of effective presentation.

READY

- You know your audience?
- You have identified 2 or 3 key messages?
- You have identified how you are going to start to grab their attention?

- You have identified how you are going to end the presentation?
- You have developed stories to help with start, end, and key points?
- You have prepared short and simple power point presentation and its script?
- You have prepared answers for probable questions?

SET

- You have considered abandoning PowerPoint all together?
- If using PowerPoint have you reduced number of slides?
- You have used pictures as well as limited text?
- Everything on your slides caters for your audience?
- You have identified where you can mix your presentation up by asking the audience questions, use of video or props and doing something unexpected?

GO

- You have practiced enough?
- You have written out notes if you need them?
- You have visualized success?
- You have asked if a lapel microphone is available?
- You made eye contact during presentation?
- You looked for the reassuring smiling faces?
- You used the techniques of both pacing and staying still?
- You satisfied the queries and cleared doubts?
- You are satisfied with yourself?

APPENDIX 1

Funding Agencies

Table 1 Major funding agencies

Funding Agency	Types of Grant	Website
University Grant Commission (UGC)	• STRIDE • Special international joint projects • Research fellowship in nonprofessional Science subjects • Junior Research fellowship in Engineering and Technology • Research award for regular University teachers	www.ugc.ac.in http://stride.bhu.ac.in/
All India Council of Technical Education (AICTE)	• Research Promotion Scheme (RPS) • MODROB • Career award for Young Scientists • National Doctoral Fellowship (NDF)	www.aicte-india.org

Table 1 *Contd...*

Funding Agency	Types of Grant	Website
Department of Science and Technology (DST)	• Core research grant • Women scientist program • Fast Track scheme for Young Scientists • IMPRINT • Bilateral international research projects • Swarna Jayanti Fellowships	www.dst.gov.in https://www.serbonline.in
Department of Biotechnology (DBT)	• Major/ minor research projects • Bilateral international projects	www.dbtindia.nic.in https://www.dbtepromis.nic.in/Login.aspx
Department of AYUSH	• Literary Research • Clinical Research	www.indianmedicine.nic.in/
Indian council of Medical Research (ICMR)	• Short Term Visiting Fellowships • Ad-hoc Research Schemes • Research Fellowships/ Associateships	www.**icmr**.nic.in

Directory of Major Journals

Journal's name	Website
AAPS PharmSci	www.aapspharmsci.org
AAPS PharmSciTech	www.aapspharmscitech.org
Acta Pharmaceutica	http://www.vnovak.hr/acphee/
Advanced Drug Delivery Reviews	http://www.elsevier.com/locate/issn/0169409X
Biological & Pharmaceutical Bulletin	http://bpb.pharm.or.jp/
Bioorganic & Medicinal Chemistry Letters	http://www.elsevier.com/locate/bmcl
Biopharmaceutics & Drug Disposition	http://www.interscience.wiley.com/jpages/0142-2782/
British Journal of Clinical Pharmacology	http://www.blackwellpublishing.com/journal.asp?ref=0306-5251
British Journal of Pharmacology	http://www.brjpharmacol.org/
Cardiovascular Drug Reviews	http://www.nevapress.com/cdr/home.html
Chemical & Pharmaceutical Bulletin	http://cpb.pharm.or.jp/
Current Pharmaceutical Biotechnology	http://www.bentham.org/cpb/index2.html

Table *Contd...*

Journal's name	Website
Current Pharmaceutical Design	http://www.bentham.org/cpd/index.html
Current Topics in Medicinal Chemistry	http://www.bentham.org/cpd/index.html
Drug Delivery	http://www.tandf.co.uk/journals/titles/10717544.asp
Drug Development and Industrial Pharmacy	http://www.dekker.com/servlet/product/productid/DDC
Drug Development Research	http://www.interscience.wiley.com/jpages/0272-4391/
Drug Discovery Today	http://www.elsevier.com/locate/issn/13596446
Expert Opinion on Drug Delivery	www.expertopine.com/eodd
Expert Opinion on Drug Discovery	www.expertopine.com/eodc
European Journal of Clinical Pharmacology	http://www.springerlink.com/openurl.asp?genre=journal&issn=0031-6970
European Journal of Medicinal Chemistry	http://www.elsevier.com/locate/issn/02235234
European Journal of Pharmaceutical Sciences	http://www.elsevier.com/locate/issn/09280987
European Journal of Pharmaceutics and Biopharmaceutics	http://www.elsevier.com/locate/issn/09396411
European Journal of Pharmacology	http://www.elsevier.com/locate/issn/00142999
Fitoterapia	http://www.elsevier.com/locate/issn/0367326X
Indian Drugs	www.indiandrugsjournal.com
Indian Journal of Pharmacology	http://www.ijp-online.com
Indian Journal of Pharmaceutical Sciences	www.ijpsonline.com
International Journal of Pharmaceutical Sciences and nanotechnology	www.ijpsnonline.com
International Journal of Pharmaceutics	http://www.elsevier.com/locate/issn/03785173
Journal of Pharmacy and Pharmacology	http://www.pharmpress.com/jpp.
International Journal of Pharmacology	www.scialert.net
Journal of Pharmacy and Pharmaceutical Sciences	http://www.ualberta.ca/~csps/Journals/JPPS.htm
Journal of Controlled Release	www.elsevier.com/journal/jcr
Journal of Microencapsulation	http://informahealthcare.com/loi/mnc
Korean Journal of Medicinal Chemistry	http://journal.kcsnet.or.kr/kcs/bkcs/bkcs_index.htm

Table *Contd...*

Journal's name	Website
Medicinal Research Reviews	http://www.interscience.wiley.com/jpages/0198-6325
Nature	http://www.nature.com/nature/
Natural Product Radiance	www.niscair.res.in
Pharmaceutical Biology	www.tandf.co.uk
Pharmaceutical Chemistry Journal	http://www.kluweronline.com/issn/0091-150X/contents
Pharmaceutical Development and Technology	http://www.dekker.com/servlet/product/productid/PDT
Pharmaceutical Research	http://www.kluweronline.com/issn/0724-8741/contents
Pharmacognosy Reviews	www.phcogrev.net
Pharmacognosy Magazine	www.phcogmag.net
Pharmacognosy Journal	www.phcog.net
Pharmacological Research	http://www.elsevier.com/locate/issn/10436618
Pharmacological Reviews	http://pharmrev.aspetjournals.org/
Pharma Review	http://www.kppub.com/
Pharmaceutical Technology	www.pharmtech .com
Phytochemical Analysis	http://mc.manuscriptcentral.com/pca
Phytomedicine	www.elsevier.com/locate/phytomed
Phytochemistry	www.ees.elsevier.com/phytochem
Planta Medica	http://www.ga-online.org/plmedica.htm
Toxicology	www.elsevier.com/locate/issn/0300483X
Tropical Journal of Pharmaceutical Research	http://www.bioline.org.br/pr
Yakugaku Zasshi / *Journal of the Pharmaceutical Society of Japan*	http://yakushi.pharm.or.jp/
The Pharmaceutical Journal	http://www.pjonline.com/Index.html

Directory of Analytical Service Providers

Service provider	Website
Indian Institute of Technology Roorkee	www.iitr.ac.in
Indian Institute of Technology Mumbai	www.iitb.ac.in
Indian Institute of Technology Kanpur	www.iitk.ac.in
Indian Institute of Technology Khargpur	www.**iit**kgp.ernet.in
Indian Institute of Technology Chennai	www.iitc.ac.in
Central Instrument Lab, Hamdard University, Delhi	http://jamiahamdard.edu/UserPanel/DisplayPage.aspx?page=eg
SAIF-Central Drug research laboratory (CDRI) Lucknow	http://www.saiflucknow.org/ www.cdriindia.org
UGC-DAE consortium for scientific research Kolkata	http://www.csr.res.in/csr/kolkata/kolkata.html

Table *Contd...*

Service provider	Website
UGC-DAE consortium for scientific research Mumbai	http://www.csr.res.in/csr/mumbai/crs.html
UGC-DAE consortium for scientific research Indore	http://www.csr.ernet.in/
UGC-DAE consortium for scientific research Kalpakkam	http://www.csr.ernet.in/csr/kalpakkam/
NIPER, Mohali	www.niper.ac.in
Western Regional Instrumentation Centre, Mumbai, Mumbai University	www.wric.mu.ac.in/
Inter University Accelerator Centre New Delhi	http://www.iuac.ernet.in/indexlowres.html
University Science Instrumentation Centre, University of Delhi	http://www.du.ac.in/index.php?id=114

E-Resources on Paper Writing

Description	Website
UGC (Promotion of Academic Integrity and Prevention of Plagiarism In Higher Educational Institutions) Regulations	https://www.ugc.ac.in/pdfnews/7771545_academic-integrity-Regulation2018.pdf
UGC'S Guidance Document "Good Academic Research Practices	https://www.ugc.ac.in/e-book/UGC_GARP_2020_Good%20Academic%20Research%20Practices.pdf
5. API Scoring: UGC Regulations on Minimum Qualification for	https://www.ugc.ac.in/pdfnews/4033931_UGC-Regulation_min_Qualification_Jul2018.pdf
appointment of Teachers and Other Academic Staff in Universities and Colleges and Measures for the Maintenance of Standards in Higher Education 2018	

Table *Contd...*

Description	Website
UGC-CARE Reference List of Quality Journals	https://ugccare.unipune.ac.in/apps1/home/index
e-PG Pathshala	www.epgp.inflibnet.ac.in
Free lectures on Academic writing	https://cutt.ly/OKlive
Author's Online Courses	https://pharmastate.academy/profile/ajaysemalty/
Academic Writing's Open Podcasting Service	http://bit.do/awpodcastsemalty
Academic Writing MOOC	www.swayamhnbgu.in
CH15 SWAYAM Prabha IIT Madras	https://www.youtube.com/channel/UC3LYjJBtm mUsC2t-VlcCkJw

Important Software for Research and Writing

Plagiarism Detection Software

Software	License	Link
Copyscape	Freemium	http://copyscape.com/
Grammarly	Freemium	https://www.grammarly.com/
HelioBLAST	Free	https://helioblast.heliotext.com/
iThenticate	Proprietary	https://www.ithenticate.com/
PrePostSEO	Freemium	https://www.prepostseo.com/plagiarism-checker
PlagiarismCheckerX	Proprietary	https://plagiarismcheckerx.com/
PlagScan	Limited	https://www.plagscan.com/en/
PlagTracker	Freemium	https://www.plagtracker.com/
ProWritingAid	Proprietary	https://prowritingaid.com/en/App/PlagiarismChecker
Turnitin	Proprietary	https://www.turnitin.com/
Unicheck	Proprietary	https://unicheck.com/
Urkund	Proprietary	https://www.urkund.com/

Grammar Correction Tools

Software	Link
Ginger Software	https://www.gingersoftware.com/
Grammar Slammer	http://englishplus.com/
Grammar Check	https://www.grammarcheck.net/
Grammarly	https://www.grammarly.com/
Hemingway Editor	http://hemingwayapp.com/
Language Tool	https://languagetool.org/
Linguix	https://linguix.com/
Paper Rater	https://www.paperrater.com/
Pro Writing Aid	https://prowritingaid.com/
Reverso	https://grammar.reverso.net/
Scribens	https://www.scribens.com/
Spell Check Plus	https://spellcheckplus.com/
WhiteSmoke	http://www.whitesmoke.com/
Writer	http://qordoba.com/

Statistical Software

Software	Developer	Link	Licence Type
GraphPad Prism	GraphPad Software, Inc.	https://www.graphpad.com/	Proprietary
Origin	OriginLab	https://www.originlab.com/	Proprietary
R	R Foundation	https://www.r-project.org/	GNU GPL
SPSS	IBM	https://www.ibm.com/products/spss-statistics	Proprietary
Statistica	Tibco Software	https://www.statistica.com/en/	Proprietary
MATLAB	MathWorks	https://mathworks.com/	Proprietary
JMP	SAS Institute	https://www.jmp.com/en_in/home.html	Proprietary

Chemical Structure Drawing Software

Software	Developer	Link	Licence Type
Avogadro	Avogadro Chemistry	https://avogadro.cc/	GNU GPL
ACD/Chem Sketch	Advanced Chemistry Development, Inc	https://www.acdlabs.com	Freemium
Chem Doodle	iChemLabs, LLC	https://www.chemdoodle.com/	Proprietary
ChemAxon	ChemAxon Ltd	https://chemaxon.com/	Proprietary
ChemDraw	PerkinElmer	https://www.perkinelmer.com	Proprietary